THE
PSYCHOLOGY
OF COVID-19

SAGE SWIFTS SERIES

The **SAGE SWIFTS** series showcases the best of social science research that has the potential to influence public policy and practice, resulting in positive social change. We strongly believe that the social sciences are uniquely positioned to make this impact and thus benefit society in a myriad of ways.

SAGE SWIFTS celebrate and support the impact of quality empirical work that provides a provocative intervention into current debates, helping society to meet critical challenges going forward.

TITLES IN THE SERIES INCLUDE:

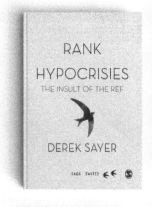

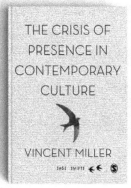

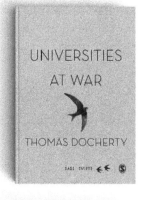

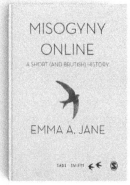

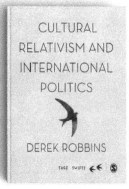

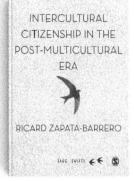

THE PSYCHOLOGY OF COVID-19

BUILDING RESILIENCE FOR FUTURE PANDEMICS

JOEL VOS

SAGE SWIFTS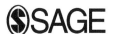

Los Angeles | London | New Delhi
Singapore | Washington DC | Melbourne

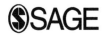

Los Angeles | London | New Delhi
Singapore | Washington DC | Melbourne

SAGE Publications Ltd
1 Oliver's Yard
55 City Road
London EC1Y 1SP

SAGE Publications Inc.
2455 Teller Road
Thousand Oaks, California 91320

SAGE Publications India Pvt Ltd
B 1/I 1 Mohan Cooperative Industrial Area
Mathura Road
New Delhi 110 044

SAGE Publications Asia-Pacific Pte Ltd
3 Church Street
#10-04 Samsung Hub
Singapore 049483

© Joel Vos 2021

First published 2021

Editor: Natalie Aguilera
Assistant editor: Eve Williams
Production editor: Sushant Nailwal
Copyeditor: Peter Williams
Indexer: Cathryn Pritchard
Marketing manager: George Kimble
Cover design: Wendy Scott
Typeset by: C&M Digitals (P) Ltd, Chennai, India

Library of Congress Control Number: 2020945813

British Library Cataloguing in Publication data

A catalogue record for this book is available from the British Library

ISBN 978-1-5297-5180-2
eISBN 978-1-5297-5206-9

To those struggling with the risks and uncertainties of pandemics, To those facing the certainties of illness or death, To those transforming the World Risk Society into a World Resilience Society.

CONTENTS

LIST OF TABLES

ABOUT THE AUTHOR

Dr. Joel Vos PhD MSc MA CPsychol FHEA. Joel is a psychologist, philosopher, researcher, public speaker and existential therapist. He is Senior Researcher at the Metanoia Institute and Research Coordinator at the New School of Psychotherapy and Counselling in London. He is a frequently asked speaker at professional conferences and public events. He chairs the IMEC International Meaning Community, such as weekly IMEC Support Groups 'MentalHealth4All', regular IMEC workshops and training, monthly IMEC Art & Music events, and annual IMEC International Meaning Conferences, During the pandemic, the IMEC support groups and conference specifically focused on coping with COVID-19. Joel has published over 100 academic articles and chapters, and has conducted and supervised many research projects. His recent research includes systematic reviews and surveys on the perception and psychological impact of the COVID-19 pandemic.

His reviews and research on meaning in life led to the publication of the books *Meaning in Life: An Evidence-based Handbook for Practitioners* (Palgrave Macmillan, 2019) and *The Economics of Meaning in Life: From Capitalist Life Syndrome to Meaning-Oriented Society* (University Professors Press, 2020). Joel's public events have led to the writing of a book together with Ron Roberts, James Davies and Psychologists for Social Change. This book, *Mental Health in Crisis,* describes the impact of modern society and politics on mental health and mental health-care (Sage, 2019).

THE WORLD RISK SOCIETY

Crisis! Chaos! Confusion! This is COVID-19: a tiny enemy that has put the world in the largest crisis for generations. With its sheer size of 0.00012 millimetres, the SARS-CoV2 virus has created significant disruption around the globe. It has made many patients gasp for air, and many health-care workers cry for more hospital beds and personal protective equipment. This virus has held almost four billion people in more than 100 countries in the chokehold of nationwide lockdowns. Economies have fallen on their knees, with gross national products and stock markets tumbling deep down. 'The new normal' AC, After COVID-19, has replaced our old lives, BC, Before COVID-19.

The world has not merely been put into crisis by this microscopic virus, but also by a larger enemy: ourselves. If COVID-19 is the first pandemic, this is the second pandemic: the psychological and political perceptions and responses to the risks and uncertainties posed by COVID-19. The psychological impact is often more extensive than the direct somatic effects of pandemics (Desclaux et al., 2017). More people may die from the lockdown than from COVID-19, due to psychological stress, lack of physical exercise and social connections, and postponing of non-COVID-19-related medical consultations and surgeries (DHSC, ONS, GAD & HO, 2020; VanderWeele, 2020). The year 2020 may also see approximately 300,000 extra suicides world-wide due to the quarantine and the subsequent economic crisis (Vos, 2020a). The psychological pandemic also seems to have made some individuals shiver in fear behind the closed curtains of their lockdown, whereas others dance their fear away at pandemic parties.

As a psychologist and philosopher, I have learned many models and tools to cope with infectious or life-threatening physical diseases (Vos, 2016). For example, when I became ill with meningitis-like symptoms in 2006 during an epidemic in an African region where I had been working, the virologist told me that I had three options: 'death, chemotherapy, or a miraculous natural recovery', – I 'chose' the third option. Although I felt frightened, I could get some sense of certainty by reading medical literature which told me about the stages of the virus. I had a roadmap of how to understand and cope with the disease. However, this time it seems different: COVID-19 does not have a clear roadmap like previous pandemics, but instead, this pandemic seems to lead us to unexpected intersections and side-tracks without knowing where we are. Yes, of course, we have a general sense of where we are coming from – from viral bats in Wuhan and the global spread of the virus – we can identify the main symptoms and the most vulnerable individuals, and we have the general direction of a vaccine in the future. However, at this moment, we are for example still unsure about the long-term symptoms, the best treatment options, the most effective precautions to minimise viral transmission, and the feasibility of developing a vaccination that will halt the pandemic. We seem to enter more unknown areas when we look at the broader social and political landscape, and at the psychological impact on individual lives. As a COVID-19 patient told me: 'We are in the Wild West.'

When the pandemic started, I brushed the dust off my health psychology models and tried to fit our collective events into these roadmaps. However, the more events I tried to fit into my models, the less I was doing justice to them. There does not seem to be a perfectly fitting model or explanation for this pandemic and how we respond to it; the only certainty is that there will be uncertainty. Uncertainties are at the heart of most pandemics and of how people respond to it – like people were uncertain what was going on and what they could do during the HIV pandemic in the 1980s. During pandemics, it seems very tempting to tell a story of certainties, and by that to create the illusion that we live in a completely safe, explainable, and controllable world – but this is not the full reality. We have to create a new roadmap, that extends our existing knowledge and helps us to understand where we are and where we could go to. This book is the reflection of my journey of exploring and mapping the uncertainties. I invite you as a companion on this journey from the known to the unknown territories. Let me introduce you to the compasses that I will use on my route in this book (see Table 1.1).

World Risk Society: The first pandemic is about epidemiological and biomedical risks. These are the risks that individuals transmit the virus, the risks that it creates severe symptoms, and the risks that it could kill people. These are risks, not facts. A risk is a chance or probability that a person will be harmed or experience adverse health effects if exposed to a hazard – in this case, SARS-CoV-2. Any specific individual could get ill but could also stay healthy. The pandemic

Table 1.1   Overview of the perspectives of this book

Perspective	Description	Example
Pandemic type	We can focus on the epidemiological and biomedical side of the COVID-19 pandemic, but we could also focus on the psychosocial and political side.	This book will not merely discuss the epidemiological and biomedical pandemic ('The First Pandemic'), but also psychosocial and political sides ('The Second Pandemic').
World Risk Society	Pandemics involve many uncertainties, such as probability calculations of infection rates and mortality rates. These calculated risks involve some amount of uncertainty, and different individuals can perceive and respond differently to these risks.	Sociologists have argued that we live nowadays in a World Risk Society, in which we are hyperconnected and exposed to many risks. Although risks involve gradients on a grey scale, individuals often seem to have black-or-white perceptions and responses to the world risk society: either they deny that any risks exist and continue living in their habitual ways, or they feel overwhelmed by the risks, develop panic and engage in obsessive-compulsive self-protection. These black-or-white perceptions and responses may have large consequences for the physical, mental and social well-being of individuals, and for the epidemiological risks and the economy in general.
Key actors	Different individuals perceive, communicate and respond differently to the risks and uncertainties of the pandemic.	This book will discuss the following key players: politicians; science; individuals experiencing stress and mental health problems; media; individuals impacted by existential threats, quarantine, and inequality.
Virus type	Pandemics can have different causes and can cause different medical diseases/symptoms	This book will discuss COVID-19 in the context of SARS, MERS, Ebola, Zika, HIV, H1N1, H5N1, and other pandemics.
Evidence	Strength of empirical evidence, e.g. conspiracy theories versus systematic research reviews	This book is based on systematic literature reviews and meta-analyses.
Resilience	Individuals and groups can be at risk, but they can also become resilient against risks.	This book will offer examples of resilience for each of the themes and will describe the World Resilience Society.
Diversity of voices	Pandemics are not merely theoretical but also involve the subjectively lived experience of individuals.	This book will exemplify the themes with citations from interviews with individuals affected by the COVID-19 pandemic.

could spiral down towards an apocalypse, be a storm in a glass of water, or be anything in between. Politicians had to make the best possible guesses, communicate the best possible information, and impose the best possible health policies, even though they had to base their perceptions and responses on unknowns and statistical probabilities.

Risks involve uncertainties: We do not know the conclusive answers and definitive solutions. There is still much unclear how we precisely got here, what is going on, and what the future could bring. This is the second pandemic: how do people perceive and respond to uncertainties? How do people perceive uncertainties, and how do they respond to the only certainty we have: the certainty of uncertainties? How do people cope with the fact that we do not live in small-scale isolated communities where everything seems pre-determined, full of certainties and habits, but we live in a hyperconnected world full of uncertainties that sociologists call the World Risk Society? Although risks involve gradients on a greyscale, individuals often seem to have black-or-white perceptions and responses to the World Risk Society: either they deny that any risks exist and they try to sustain their habitual lifestyle, or they feel overwhelmed by the risks, panic and engage in obsessive-compulsive self-protection and stockpiling. These black-or-white perceptions and responses may impact their physical, mental, and social well-being, and could influence the progression of the pandemic and the economic depression. This fundamental question that this book seeks to answer is: how much uncertainty can society bear? How much uncertainty can we live with as individuals? How can we transform meaningless uncertainties into meaningful opportunities to live a meaningful and satisfying life together, despite the risks surrounding us? How can we prevent powerful individuals from using the uncertainties to their advantage and to the disadvantage of the public?

Key actors: To understand the psychology of COVID-19 is to understand how individuals perceive and respond to the uncertainties of the World Risk Society. However, we need to differentiate uncertainties in different life domains, which each have their own key actors (Vos, 2011). First Nation Canadians have been telling us for more than 10,000 years that we could identify three life domains, which connect like a circle inside a circle (Vos, 2020). The outer circle is about the universe, the world and nature in which we live. This is where we will start our journey. In modern societies, scientists are usually the people who tell us what is going on here; therefore I will explore how scientists describe the risks of nature, and how they cope with their own uncertainties (Chapter 2). The middle circle, which sits within the outer circle, is about society and community. Of course, we will start to investigate the social risks, and how politicians perceive these and how they cope with their own uncertainties (Chapter 3). Nevertheless, they are not the only leading figures in society; there are many other high-status people, journalists, and social influencers. Therefore, we will describe the role of traditional and social media (Chapter 4). The most inner circle is about ourselves. We need to start examining how we look at these other circles around us. For example, how do individuals perceive scientific risks? How do they perceive and get influenced by the certainties and uncertainties presented by politicians and media? Therefore, we will examine individual risk-perception (Chapter 5). This risk-perception does not function as a hard border between the self and the social and natural world; no, the risk-perception influences how we feel about the risks and uncertainties that the world around us pose on us. Therefore, we will subsequently analyse the impact of the pandemic, and our perception of it, on our mental health (Chapter 6). Our existential position sits in the core of the circular model, describing our approach to life, and how we cope with the existential threat of COVID-19. What is our most fundamental position in life towards uncertainties: do we try to push them away, or do we authentically acknowledge them and transform them into opportunities to live a meaningful and satisfying life (Chapter 7)? After this journey that started at the outer ring of nature and science and that ended with our existential attitude towards life, only one question remains: do we still want to live in the World Risk Society? Or do we want to transform this into a World Resilience Society, where risks become opportunities? What would such a World Resilience Society look like? What would this mean for how we cope with the COVID-19 pandemic and with future pandemics (Chapter 8)?

World Resilience Society: This book ultimately offers hope and calls for action. We can – and possibly should? – change our perception and responses to the World Risk Society, to build resilience for future pandemics. Resilience is the capacity to adjust to challenges flexibly and to recover quickly from difficulties, like a young twig on a tree is resilient as it can withstand storms whereas an old rigid branch may crack. The last chapters will offer glimpses of hope for coping in more resilient ways with future pandemics, and these will lay out how we could move from a World Risk Society to a World Resilience Society. Nevertheless, before we can build a new society on new foundations – or rebuild old collapsed buildings – we need to know where our current weaknesses are and why our current society has failed, as we will see in the first chapters of this book.

Virus type: Let us start with the official story from the World Health Organisation, although alternative theories are circulating on the fringes of scientific literature. Pandemics are large-scale epidemics afflicting people across the globe, caused by organisms – bacteria or viruses – for which most people do not have pre-existing immunity, and which can transmit easily between individuals and lead to severe disease (WHO.int, 10/09/2020). This book will focus on the new coronavirus which initially emerged in the Chinese region of Wuhan at the end of 2019, and which quickly spread globally: SARS-CoV-2. This virus can lead to respiratory illness with symptoms such as fever, coughing, sore throat, shortness of breath and sometimes a lack of taste and smell, and cardiovascular symptoms. Eighty per cent of all patients experience mild symptoms, whereas 13% experience severe symptoms and 6% suffer from critical conditions such as severe pneumonia and respiratory or multiple organ failure. Whereas most patients experience these symptoms only for a brief period, almost one in five report remaining symptoms in the long term. Individuals most at risk of developing severe COVID-19 are elderly individuals and those with underlying medical conditions (Emami et al., 2020; Sun et al., 2020). COVID-19 is the third large coronavirus outbreak in less than 20 years, after the Severe Acute Respiratory Syndrome (SARS) in 2002–3 and the Middle East Acute Respiratory Syndrome (MERS) in 2012. Other recent pandemics include the Zika virus in 2015, the H1N1 swine flu in 2009, the H5N1 bird flu in 2008, and the Ebola virus in 2004. As there is still much unknown about the treatment of the biomedical characteristics and the psychological impact of COVID-19, this book will also use the findings from these other pandemics.

Evidence: It seems easy to fall into Big Conspiracy Theories, but much harder to critically use empirical science. The COVID-19 pandemic seems to have thrown the scientific method from its pedestal – again – and replaced this with Key Influencers on social media. However, this is not an either-or story: either we totally trust science, or we trust Conspiracy Theorists. I will critically interpret the findings of empirical research and acknowledge its limitations while underlining the uncertainties. For example, I will describe how science in times of pandemics is extraordinary science, focused on making quick decisions based on uncertainties – we cannot completely generalise science in these times with usual academic processes. This uncertain science may lead to uncertain politics, with illogical jumps in reasoning and unjustified conclusions and recommendations for public health. We can criticise these uncertain sciences and policies by using research against research. This book is grounded in systematic critical reviews of empirical research; rigorous analyses of COVID-19 are needed to separate the wheat from the chaff, and not merely base conclusions and recommendations on single studies, opinions, or hypes.

Diversity of voices: Pandemics are not merely about theories but involve the subjectively lived experiences of individuals. Therefore, this book will include the lived experiences of individuals and not merely theoretical essays. Let me introduce some of the twenty individuals who I have interviewed for this book. My negotiations with them about these interviews provide another example of the Second Pandemic, as they only agreed to be interviewed if I used pseudonyms since, they told me, they could be fired or even legally prosecuted if it became known that they had been blowing the whistle. The necessity for this secrecy is telling: managers and health authorities seem to be wanting to cast out any uncertainties, and present their perfect story full of certainties. It is this story of uncertainties that I want to tell in this book: the story of the Second Pandemic.

'When this pandemic is over, I will leave my work as a nurse. I cannot work anymore with these lies and the lack of equipment from this government… and of course with the utter disorganisation of the National Health Services.' (Emma, Intensive care unit nurse)

'Even though it is now six months since the initial diagnosis, and all my CT scans and blood tests are fine, I am still exhausted; will I ever be better again? My friends and family still avoid me like the plague; will I ever be trusted again? It feels as if my body is in a big fight. On most days, I keep going because I am hoping that scientists will develop a treatment and vaccine. On other days, I do not have the energy and I just want to surrender and let COVID-19 take my life.' (Richard, COVID-19 patient)

'The COVID-19 numbers did initially not add up – there is a serious flu going on, but no pandemic. When I told my manager, he threatened to fire me.' (Martin, biomedical data analyst)

'On day one, we were told that there is a pandemic. On day five, our shop had to close the doors. On day ten, I was made redundant. Around day thirty, I could not pay my rent anymore.' (Peter, unemployed, after losing his job in retail)

2

NATURAL RISKS

UNCERTAIN SCIENCE

'Scientists do not really do certainty. All of science is based around the models that we construct to tell us about the things we are interested in, and the experiments that we conduct to see whether the models match the reality on the ground. It is this combination of model and experiment, trial and error and correction, that help us understand the world.' (Dobson, 2020: 3)

OVERVIEW OF PANDEMIC SCIENCE

On a grey, cloudy day in March 2020, a young data analyst was staring at the numbers on his screen. He mumbled to himself: 'This cannot be right!' His spreadsheet showed three columns, with written on the top 'positive test-result', 'negative test-result' and 'no-test'; the rows displayed the hospital numbers of patients. He shook his head and picked up his phone, selecting the contact number of his colleague.

'Hi, Martin here. Would you have a minute? I am now looking at the figures, but I can only find a moderately strong relationship between mortality and a positive test result for COVID-19. There does not seem to be a large pandemic going on here.'

A brief silence followed, followed by Martin saying: 'So you are saying that we may explain this lack of correlation by the lack of specificity and sensitivity of the tests? There are too many uncertainties about these test results?'

Martin hummed in agreement with the speaker. 'Yes, I have also calculated that. I did not use a positive test result as the criterion of "COVID-19 death", but instead used the presence of any physical symptoms associated with COVID-19, such as sudden high fever, a new continuous cough or respiratory disease. This time, I found a significant correlation between these symptoms and mortality, but I do not feel certain about these analyses, as we do not know whether these symptoms can be attributed to COVID-19. Of course, this dataset is more complete than the one based on positive COVID-19 tests, as we have more detailed information about the symptoms of patients, as not everyone has had a COVID-19 test. But ultimately, both statistical models are full of uncertainties, both the one based on a positive test result and the one on physical symptoms.'

Martin frowned and looked puzzled when his colleague spoke. 'What are you saying? Should I compare the current mortality figure with the figures from last year? How do we know that these excess deaths are due to COVID-19? They could also be due to the side-effects of the lockdown, such as the closure of hospital departments – many patients missed crucial surgeries or check-ups, for example for cancer or cardiovascular disease. This statistical model will be similarly full of uncertainties.'

After the phone conversation, the young data analyst sat down in silence, holding his head in his hands. What statistical model is the best? Which model has the least uncertainties? There does not seem to be any perfect model. He can estimate the statistical likelihood for each model, but all of these will be estimations. Hard science seems impossible.

Martin told me about his struggles with the continuous changes in the dictates from health authorities about the ways in which patient data were collected and analysed. He explained that different models lead to different conclusions about infection rates and mortality rates. Each model is based on different hypotheses, such as the sensitivity of a test to identify COVID-19 in a patient who actually has COVID, and the specificity to not give a positive test result for patients who are not ill. While the pandemic was unfolding, there were many uncertainties and there was a lack of sufficient sensitive and specific tests for adequate monitoring and statistical predicting. Martin described how he felt many – often conflicting – pressures on him by his managers and the governmental Department of Health. There was no certainty. There was no clear paradigm. The only thing he was certain about was uncertainty, and he told me how different people would try to mold the uncertain figures into certainties which were not there, such as concluding that there is either a massive pandemic or a total absence of a crisis. He described that the science during pandemics is uncertain, even though the uncertainties may be transformed into certainties by higher powers.

This book has to start with science and data, and the uncertainties surrounding these. The political decisions, the public debate, the media, and the individual psychological impact all start with the information from scientists. To understand the psychology of COVID-19 means understanding how scientists make decisions in uncertain times, and how these uncertainties are communicated to the broader population, and how individual citizens develop their theories about the pandemic. In this chapter, I will describe the psychology behind the decision-making of researchers, governments, health-care providers, pharmaceutical companies, and international institutions such as the WHO. This will show that research during the pandemic stands on three shaky foundations: the lack of preparedness of the health services, the inaccuracy of data collection, and the influence of powerful individuals and companies on how the data are interpreted and used for large-scale measures. Several examples will follow, such as the debates regarding herd immunity and nationwide lockdown.

Table 2.1 A psychological approach to pandemic science

Psychological mode	Description	COVID-19 example
Non-paradigmatic science	Science during pandemics functions differently than during normal times, as it involves many uncertainties about data, methods and models, while health authorities need to make quick decisions on the basis of this uncertain information.	Different health authorities have used different models at different times to calculate infection rates and mortality rates.
Academic crisis	Academic research seems to have less authoritative status in society than in the past. This may be due to postmodernism, popularisation and financial dependence.	On social media, laypeople discuss scientific research, and social media influencers and alternative scientists seem to receive much attention.
Governmental decision-making	Governments and health authorities often make decisions not in a rational way, but slowly muddle-through in incremental steps, with powerful individuals dominating the decisions. Executive powers seem to have a more determining role, and some decisions seem to be made for the main purpose of political propaganda.	The British House of Lords and the American Senate have started investigations into the decision-making processes and accountability during the COVID-19 pandemic.

Psychological mode	Description	COVID-19 example
Pharmaceutical companies	Pharmaceutical companies are an important economic and political power and can influence scientific conclusions and political decisions via lobbying and trade deals.	The WHO announcement that there is a pandemic automatically activated trade deals between governments and pharmaceutical companies. Big Pharma has invested in lobbying for new deals.
International institutions	Global health is monitored and influenced by multi-country institutions such as the WHO and private-public partnerships. Communication by these institutions is very influential in determining the strategies of states. Most R&D funding goes to specific diseases and pandemics, and not to building basic structural health-care. There have been criticisms over a lack of transparency over decision-making, and over commercial and pharmaceutical influences on decisions.	In response to failures during previous pandemics, the WHO has developed sensitive warning systems and R&D mechanisms which were quickly activated with the first signs of the COVID-19 pandemic.

Table 2.2 Applications of the psychological approach to pandemic science

Application	Description	COVID-19 example
Lack of preparedness	Scientists have been warning states for decades about the increased likelihood of pandemics, and have recommended them to prepare for pandemics (e.g. buy sufficient PPE and ventilators).	Several states seemed relatively unprepared to cope with the pandemic (e.g. lack of PPE and ventilators), as consecutive governments have decided not to allocate sufficient resources. If they were prepared, they often focused on the worst-case scenario, and not on relatively mild diseases.
Uncertain data	Data are regarded as essential to monitor the development of pandemics, and to use as foundations of health policies.	Different health authorities have used different models at different times to calculate infection rates and mortality rates.

(Continued)

Table 2.2   (Continued)

Application	Description	COVID-19 example
Herd immunity	Politicians have debated the option to let people catch the virus so that they build antibodies which could stop the pandemic.	During the COVID-19 pandemic, there was insufficient information about the building of antibodies and the impossibility to get a second infection. The public debate also seemed to sketch this option as immoral.
Nationwide lockdown	Countries have been put into a lockdown to protect individuals from spreading the virus and to prevent health services being overwhelmed by too many patients for whose treatment they lack sufficient resources. Prior to the pandemic, there was little empirical evidence for the effects of nationwide lockdowns, and the main decisions for lockdown were made on the basis of theoretical and simplified mathematical models.	More than 4 billion individuals in over 100 countries have been in lockdown. It has been estimated that the side effects of the lockdown may have led to mortality figures about half the size of the COVID-19 mortality figures, and some scientists have sketched effects larger than the pandemic.

NON-PARADIGMATIC SCIENCE

Science during pandemics is extraordinary science, as researchers need to make bold conclusions and brash recommendations while there are still many uncertainties:

> '[Science during a pandemic] reflects the transition between normal science and a post-normal form of managing risk.' (Abeysinghe, in Bjørkdahl & Carlsen, 2018, p.13)

We live under the dictatorship of urgency. Pandemic science is based on statistical risk calculations, not on absolute facts or the results from nationwide experiments. This reality of scientific uncertainty and extraordinary science seems to clash with the needs of the population: people want certainty, control, and clear explanations. Consequently, scientists are often the target of political and public outrage, on whom people project their frustration about the pandemic. It is this vacuum of unfulfilled hopes and dreams that self-acclaimed social media 'scientists' and conspiracy theorists attempt to fill, although it is an illusion that anyone could achieve total certainty in the early stages of a pandemic. Possibly in later stages, things may become clearer but with possibly new mutations and dynamic social contexts, even that is not sure. This is the best we can know.

The philosopher Thomas Kuhn (2012) described the history of science as normal times and revolutions. In normal times, there seems to be a relative consensus around a core set of concepts or thought patterns, including theories, research methods, postulates, and standards for what constitutes legitimate contributions to a field. He calls this model of reality that dominates science a 'paradigm'. In normal times, most scientists will do research within this existing paradigm, and any ideas that lie outside of this paradigm may be attacked by colleagues and called 'unscientific'. Consequently, uncertainties and flaws are ignored – or get reinforced – due to self-policing within the scientific community. However, a paradigm shift may occur if many critical anomalies accumulate over time, and a new theory may emerge which both encompasses older research ideas and explains relevant anomalies.

Paradigm shifts are often quite dramatic and may involve radical actions by politicians and commercial actors who may have a stake in maintaining the old paradigm. For example, when the University of Pisa was in a lockdown during a plague outbreak between 1630 and 1633, Galileo Galilei worked from his home on his theories about natural laws. The story goes that Galileo saw an apple falling from the tree in his garden, which led him to formulate the Law of Gravity and the Heliocentric Theory. As these theories went against the dominant paradigms in science and religion, the Roman Inquisition tried Galileo in 1633 and found him 'vehemently suspect of heresy', sentencing him to indefinite house arrest until he died in 1642. This sentencing reminds us of the psychological need for social structure and the biopolitical mechanism of exclusion, which can get triggered in times of collective crisis and change. However, after Galileo's arrest, new research started to accumulate, proving his theories, and in 1992 the Vatican finally vindicated him.

Similar secular ex-communications seem to be happening during COVID-19. For example, on 6 September 2020, the Council of Europe issued a formal level 2 media freedom alert over the UK government blacklisting of investigative journalists and structurally denying them access to information (*The Independent*, 06/09/2020). Furthermore, there are stories about the arrests of scientists who ask critical questions about the scientific evidence for national strategies, such as professors Li Wenliang and Chen Zhaozhi in China, Anastasia Vasilieva in Russia, and Thomas Binder in Switzerland. Social media such as Facebook and YouTube have automatically been deleting posts and profiles which they deem 'fake'. Facebook has started to inform users which posts it regards as including 'fake news', such as David Icke. The argument from these social media giants is that the voice of these agitators may prevent other people from self-isolating or using PPE. However, from a psychological perspective it is questionable how effective censorship is, for example because censorship may raise public suspicions even more and reinforce conspiracy theories (see Chapter 4). By labelling non-paradigmatic voices as 'controversial', 'uncertain', or even 'abject', these censors seem to contribute to the creation of an uncritical, self-serving authoritarian culture, which may be less effective in finding revolutionary scientific solutions to the pandemic and other societal crises. Although we may fundamentally disagree with the ideas and methods of some of these rebels – for instance because some of their methods seem questionable – their critical voices form a part of the scientific and public debate – of normal and revolutionary times of science – and censorship may undermine the democratic and healthy functioning of science.

ACADEMIC CRISIS

At the end of the 20th century, academics have lost the status they once occupied in society. Truth seems to have become interchangeable with opinion. A president wins support by tweeting his opinion against 99% of the scientific consensus on climate change. The local butcher has become an expert on epidemiology in his conversations with his customers. Of course, it can be hailed that academia has become much more democratic by making scientific ideas accessible to the broad public. However, the traditional academic elite sometimes seems to have been replaced by a new elite, one of tweeting populists and YouTube gurus. Even worse, as the following sections will elaborate, commercial powers may have been trying to buy what we consider to be the truth, and politicians may have been twisting the truth. How did academics slide down into this new role, and how does this new role influence how laypeople perceive and respond to the science about COVID-19?

Postmodernism: Modern science started in the Renaissance, with researchers conducting meticulous observations and experiments. Many scientists seemed to share the idea that there is an absolute universal truth lying in the world around us, waiting to be measured and categorised via instruments such as thermometers and micrometers. By discovering these truths, we can possibly better master our world and improve our quality of life. However, the birth of social sciences at the end of the 19th century meant an end to this modernist idea about truths: scientists are also just human beings, scientific instruments are human products, and psychological bias and social processes may influence research. Even physical experiments do not seem to provide the hard facts we had once thought: observing a physical phenomenon can change the phenomenon.

Postmodernism tells that there is not One Big Certain Story that scientists can tell about the world around us – there are only small stories by individual storytellers. All science is a human process, and all truths are relative. Similarly, there may not be one absolute truth about COVID-19, waiting to be discovered: we may only be able to scrape some observations together, create an assemblage of this relatively random selection of findings, and blow this up to a large story about the truth of COVID-19 – even though our foundations are uncertain and incommensurable findings. These assemblage and narrating processes are not absolute but can be swayed by our values and our scientific paradigm, and by political and commercial influences. This postmodern perspective can also be applied to the scientific models of pandemics:

> 'The value of modelling must therefore be recognised as conditional and partial – thus requiring attention to dialogue, deliberation and the practical politics both of conception and application. Models are about different ways of making sense, not definitive ways of asserting precise predictions. Beyond the narrow models that often define a predictive risk paradigm, there are of course alternative cultures of modelling. Here plurality is central – different models tell contrasting stories, and the key for policy is the conversation between them. Models may be derived from different sources of knowledge – from high-end science to more grounded, participatory insights – and so the story must be told as part of an interactive translation between idioms and explanations. For example, in infectious disease management, analysts may confront uncertainties emerging from process models that examine the underlying population dynamics, from pattern models that explore the spatial dimensions of disease and from participatory models rooted in local people's perspectives, as differentiated by class, age and gender. Only by developing a narrative across all three can a more integrated and effective perspective on disease control emerge.' (Scoones & Stirling, 2020, p.11)

Popularisation: Thus, in our postmodern era, academics seem to have tumbled from their societal pedestals, and have become fallible humans – like laypeople. The 1968 student riots further accelerated the democratisation process of academia, as students demanded more influence on the running of universities. This student revolution was part of a broader revolution in science, which transformed the idea that science has to be complicated and that people need to study long to understand what academics are saying. Nowadays, academic research is no longer merely justified by peer judgment of the quality of their research as it also has to connect with society: which impact does research have on society, and how do researchers engage with the public?

A side effect of this process of democratisation and increased transparency is the emergence of pop-science: the interpretation of science for the broad audience. The aims and methods of science have changed: whereas formal science aims to inform and persuade peers about the reliability, validity and trustworthiness of their observations and conclusions, often with detailed methods and nuanced formulations, popular science seems to aim at informing and convincing scientific outsiders about the relevance of the findings, often with simplifications and broad sweeping statements. Pop-science seems to have become a large profitable industry, selling science as entertainment and emphasising the uniqueness and radicalness of the findings. Newspapers, magazines, and TV shows would not sell well with dry scientists explaining detailed complex theories with unknown relevance for the audience. The pop-culture also seems to raise individual scientists to pop-heroes, like the British epidemiologist Neil Ferguson and the American national health advisor Anthony Fauci – with media publishing countless interviews and personal profiles on who they are, as if their personality matters more than their science. Thus, the public aims and methods of science seem to be almost the opposite of academic aims and methods.

Consequently, whereas academics may see a scientific study as an uncertain assemblage of relatively random findings and probability calculations, pop-science could present the same findings as a black-or-white truth or certainty. It also seems that the popularisation of science has created the expectation in the general public, that scientists can give immediate clear-cut answers and solutions for our individual daily lives, hiding the decades or centuries of research on which these pop-certainties are based. COVID-19 seems to be the apotheosis of pop-science with a broad public debate over scientific truths and 'fake news'.

Financial dependence: At the end of the 20th century, in many countries, governments have reduced the funding of universities and research. To fund their research, tuition fees have increased, universities attract as many students as possible and rent out their accommodations for high prices (Vos et al., 2019). There is pressure to patent and sell scientific discoveries to finance research institutes. Scientists have also requested commercial partners to fund their academic research and increasing numbers of researchers have left universities to join commercial laboratories. Consequently, most research – 71%, for example, in the USA – is nowadays funded by private companies, venture capitalists, philanthropists or non-profit foundations (Boroush, 2015). An increasing amount of this funding goes to innovative research, and a minority to fundamental or theoretical studies (PwC.com, Global Innovation 1000 Study).

As a consequence of this ever-increasing financial dependence on commercial grants, scientists are under pressure to deliver innovative research that can be marketised and sold for large profits. This dependence on commercial funding could make researchers consciously or unconsciously biased (Bodenheimer, 2000). A systematic review found a statistically significant association between industry sponsorship and pro-industry conclusions, and thus 'conflicts of interest arising from these ties can influence biomedical research in important ways' (Lesser et al., 2007). Science also seems biased, because usually only new and positive findings get published. Eighty-five per cent of industry-funded studies are positive, but only 50% of the government-funded trials (Bourgeois et al., 2010). The pharmaceutical industry often limits the trial design, accessing the raw data and the interpretations of the results by researchers (Davidoff et al., 2001), and pressure authors not to disclose their financial interests in any scientific publications so that it remains unclear to the reader to which extent the research may be biased (Cochrane, 2011). Almost 16% of all publicly funded researchers admit that they have altered the design, methodology or results under pressure from an external funding source (Martinson et al., 2005). One review culminated in a shocking punchline: 'The results from every Randomized Controlled Trial favoured the drug of the sponsor' (Fries & Krishnan, 2004). The epidemiologist Vandenbroucke (2006) even calls all industry-sponsored drug-trials 'not research, but marketing'. Goldacre (2013, pp. x–xi) summarises the structural problems in the following way, which does not give much trust in Big Pharma as the Superheroes who will come to our rescue during the COVID-19 pandemic:

'Drugs are tested by the people who manufacture them, in poorly designed trials, on hopelessly small numbers of weird, unrepresentative patients, and analysed using techniques which are flawed by design, in such a way that they exaggerate the benefits of treatments. Unsurprisingly, these trials tend to produce results that favour the manufacturer. When trials throw up results that companies don't like, they are perfectly entitled to hide them from doctors and patients, so we only ever see a distorted picture of any drug's true effects. Regulators see most of the trial data, but only from early on in a drug's life, and even then they don't give this data to doctors or patients, or even to other parts of the government. This distorted evidence is then communicated and applied in a distorted fashion. In their forty years of practice after leaving medical school, doctors hear about what works through ad hoc oral traditions, from sales reps, colleagues or journals. But those colleagues

can be in the pay of drug companies – often undisclosed – and the journals are too. Academic papers, which everyone thinks of as objective, are often covertly planned and written by people who work directly for the companies, without disclosure. Sometimes whole academic journals are even owned outright by one drug company. Aside from all this, for several of the most important and enduring problems in medicine, we have no idea what the best treatment is, because it's not in anyone's financial interest to conduct any trials at all. These are ongoing problems, and although people have claimed to fix many of them, for the most part they have failed; so all these problems persist, but worse than ever, because now people can pretend that everything is fine after all.'

COVID-19 Scientific Crisis: These examples of scientific corruption and fraud seem to have further undermined the public trust in science, in addition to the effects of postmodernism and pop-science. Instead of trusting scientists, non-specialists seem to progressively create their subjective assemblage of scattered observations, random research findings, and logical fallacies, leading to the popularisation of conspiracy theories as will be explained in a later chapter. Criticism of scientists and unfounded hypotheses seem rife on social media. This trend of lowered scientific standards is exacerbated by the decision of major trusts and scientific journals to make all COVID-19-related articles available for the broad public, even before peer review by peers. During the first six months of the pandemic, 100,000 more studies than usual have been published, with the majority lacking peer review (Nature Index, 2020). The public accessibility of these articles – which are often pre-published while peers and journal editors are still reviewing them – makes scientific collaboration and progress more democratic and faster. However, this also means that these publications lack the usual review before publication process which separates the wheat from the chaff. This means that the normal high standard of scientific scrutiny is absent which usually prevents low-quality studies becoming a hype in the public domain. These trends seem to exacerbate the crisis that science has already been in before the pandemic.

GOVERNMENTAL DECISION-MAKING

How are scientific findings translated into national health policies? How have governments made decisions regarding COVID-19? The following paragraphs will explain how governmental decisions are made incrementally, under the increasing influence of executive powers, and political propaganda, and how this has happened during the pandemic. Whereas we will now examine the psychology of how governments have created their policies on the basis of uncertain science, the next chapter will elaborate how these political decisions have subsequently psychologically impacted ordinary citizens.

Incremental model: Governments usually do not linearly make decisions, with a simple weighing of the pros and cons of all possible alternatives. Research shows that governmental departments usually do not follow such a rational decision-making process, because multiple departments and advisory committees are involved, and decision-makers are often limited by little time and small budgets. Consequently, making decisions is often described as 'muddling through' (Lindblom, 1959). That is, decision-makers make some steps, compare the first available alternatives, secure the agreement of key stakeholders, and then finalise a quick decision. Decisions are often also influenced by previous decisions – which is called 'path dependency' in political sciences – and by institutional stickiness due to the inertia of many stakeholders. In such slow and complex decision-making processes, it may come as a relief when lobbyists offer quick, cheap and promising short-cuts –'no worries, if you give us this contract, we can take this problem off of your shoulders'. The political post-mortem analysis of the COVID-19 pandemic by the British House of Lords Committee received similar reports of muddling through, inertia and overpowering individuals, as we will examine in more detail later in this chapter.

Executive powers takeover: Several changes have emerged in Western government decision-making processes since the 1990s (Rosanvallon, 2013). To short-cut the decision-making process, departments have reduced the number of advisory committees, or only appoint committees ad hoc. Until the 1990s, governmental departments often had semi-independent committees of researchers; however, during the global trend of Third Way politics, such as New Labour in the United Kingdom, many committees were deleted for the reason of making political decision-making faster and cheaper. In practice, this did often not result in faster and cheaper decision-making as ministers or secretaries had to ask civil servants to search for external scientists who could write reports. This process of searching for new scientists for each new governmental proposal has been described as expensive and also as biasing the outcomes of the research, as civil servants could select researchers who were likely to support the governmental proposal under study. Instead of having a balanced debate between researchers on governmental proposals, unelected top civil servants and unelected advisors have increasing monopoly powers to select the researchers and the reports they want to make publicly available, in line with the proposals of ministers or secretaries. The lack of transparency and scientific integrity seems to be aggravated by the gagging clauses in the governmental contracts with the external researchers, so that researchers cannot speak publicly about their findings even if the government decides to hide their study. These developments imply that modern government policies may not always be based on independent, systematic scientific evidence. It seems that science has often become an extension of politics.

This trend of partial outsourcing of research seems to go hand-in-hand with general growth of the executive powers. For example, Rosanvallon (2013) describes that parliaments in Western countries seem to have less power and that courts get increasingly influenced by the government – for example by the political allocation of judges and members of the Senate or the House of Lords. For example, several countries have passed COVID-19 emergency laws which immediately decreased the powers of health authorities – including the scientists and experts on pandemics – and demoted them to mere advisors, while giving large powers to non-expert governmental ministers and civil servants (e.g. Danish Parliament Proceedings, 12/03/2020). Consequently, unscientific decisions from governments can pass with relatively little legislative and judiciary scrutiny and with biased accountability procedures. Another example of this dominance of the executive power could be the COVID-19 bills and acts which seem to have been approved by parliaments with a historical fast speed, possibly without the systematic scrutiny that such revolutionary decisions would usually have received in normal times in the past.

Political propaganda: Under the influence of neoliberal think tanks, the British minister Sir Keith Joseph – the right hand of Margaret Thatcher wrote in his white and green papers that policy decisions should aim at increasing the support of voters and decreasing political opposition (Vos, 2020; Vos et al., 2019). For example, according to Joseph, education should focus more on skills that the main economic sectors need, and less on sociology and critical thinking skills which could grow political opposition. Labour 'red' neighbourhoods of council housing should be broken up by allowing the wealthiest individuals to buy their houses. Similarly, Joseph proposed the selective governmental outsourcing of research. Thus, he ultimately argued that all governmental decisions are electoral propaganda. From this perspective, the fundamental question is to what extent the governmental decisions about the pandemic may also be used as political propaganda. To answer the question about possible bias in the political decisions during the pandemic, the British House of Lords and the American Senate have started investigations into the decision-making processes and accountability during the COVID-19 pandemic. The minutes of these investigation committees make interesting reading and seem to confirm the incremental decision-making process, the monopoly of executive powers – and the dominance of specific top advisors and politicians – and electoral propaganda (e.g. Betrus, 2020; Qazi, 2020).

For example, the United Kingdom has a specific scientific committee, SAGE, which advises the government on COVID-19. Journalists have shown that SAGE members have direct ties with pharmaceutical companies who will create the vaccinations for COVID-19, a lack of experts on behavioural science and intensive care, and the presence of political advisors who veto the decisions of the SAGE committee (*The Times*, 09/05/2020; *The Guardian* 01/06/2020; *True Republica*, 01/06/2020; *Off-Guardian*, 28/05/2020; *The Independent*, 25/05/2020; *The Guardian*, 08/05/2020; *Bloomberg*, 29/04/2020). Journalists have also questioned the quality of the data on which these committees have based their research, as they have used suspect data from companies with commercial interests (*The Guardian*, 05/06/2020; *Full Fact*, 04/06/2020; OpenDemocracy, 05/06/2020).

PHARMACEUTICAL COMPANIES

Pharmaceutical companies run the world. This seems to be an unavoidable conclusion after reading books with titles such as: *Pharma* (Posner, 2020), *Deadly Medicines and Organised Crime* (Gøtzsche, 2013), *Bad Pharma* (Goldacre, 2013) and *Doubt Is Their Product* (Michaels, 2008). Research shows that the pharmaceutical industry has an annual gross income of $1 trillion, which is approximately 0.7% of global GDP (b2international.com, 10/09/2020). It is understandable that there are many critical questions and conspiracy theories about such a powerful industry. Although Big Pharma may increase their sales if a COVID-19 vaccine becomes available, some biotech experts doubt that this will provide a large profit, due to political and public pressure to keep the price low (*Investment Trust Insider*, 16/07/2020). Currently, some Big Pharma have announced vaccine prices between $3 and $35; if each person in the world were vaccinated, this would be about $133 billion gross (13% of the annual income of Big Pharma; however, the new trials indicate that two or three shots are needed for full immunity, thus doubling or tripling the expected profits).

However, pharmaceutical giants are more than their research and sales; for examples, there has been an increase of 500% in the shares of pharmaceutical companies who seem to be on course for winning the race for developing the first COVID-19 vaccine (*Bloomberg*, 20/07/2020). Thus although Big Pharma may only have relatively small profits from COVID-19 vaccines – any profits from COVID-19 treatment medication and equipment excluded – their investors seem to feel satisfied, as one newspaper wrote: 'Give your portfolio a shot in the arm... by investing in the shares of the companies working to beat coronavirus' (*Financial Mail on Sunday*, 18/04/2020). The following paragraphs offer an overview of the effects that the pharmaceutical industry has had on science and government decision-making. These influences raise critical questions about how we organise our healthcare and governments, and how governments have made decisions during COVID-19.

Unsurprisingly, a ping-pong game between critical scientists and Big Pharma immediately emerged when the UK was the first country to approve a COVID-19 vaccination at 3 December 2020. American immunologist Fauci commented that the approval procedures have been less deep compared to the the US and the past (The Independent, 3/12/2020). Scientists also launched a petition to demand more advanced and longer-lasting safety trials before vaccinations are made available to the general population, for example to exclude risks that may only become visible on long-term, such as infertility (Wodarg & Yeadon, 2020). In response, the British Prime Minister and Healthy Secretary told the press that the vaccines 'are totally safe' and that 'misinformation should be censored'; their appeal was followed by Facebook and YouTube announcing that they would 'remove COVID-19 misinformation' about this new vaccine (The Verge, 3/12/2020).

Lobbying: A frequently heard criticism is that pharmaceutical companies use – or, as some Conspiracy Theorists have argued, have even caused – the pandemic as a shock doctrine to sell treatments and vaccinations. Journalists point at evidence that pharmaceutical lobbyists have been trying to sell their products to governments – as any profit-making company would possibly do when there is a business opportunity. Pharmaceutical industries go hand-in-hand with propaganda; many companies try, for example, to influence how media portray health issues, for example via owning shares of newspapers, sharing their research reports, paying celebrities to promote their products and advertising; Big Pharma spent over $90 billion annually on advertising (Posner, 2020; Vos et al., 2019). Furthermore, several authors have argued that there is a revolving door between pharmaceutical companies and regulators (Goldacre, 2013), and the US Justice Department's antitrust division describes the secret collaborations between pharmaceutical companies 'the most pervasive and harmful criminal antitrust conspiracy ever uncovered' (*New York Times*, 10/10/1999). For example, Roche has convinced governments to stockpile the drug Tamiflu for billions – 'the biggest theft in history' – to treat seasonal flu, even though it only reduces some symptoms for a maximum of 21 hours. Will pharmaceutical companies now suddenly change and behave completely ethically during the COVID-19 pandemic?

COVID-19 trade deals: The most controversial influence from pharmaceutical industries is the pressure of Big Pharma on the WHO to remove the criterion of the disease severity to identify a pandemic; this removal means, for example, that the number of deaths is not relevant to announce a pandemic (Lakoff, 2017). The removal of this criterion has made the WHO declare COVID-19 a pandemic earlier than it might have done before. Furthermore, during the COVID-19 pandemic, the researcher Olson found together with his colleagues (2020) that pharmaceutical companies in the US have increased their lobbying expenditures ($248.4 million) and new lobbyist registrations (357), in response to the announcement of the most extensive stimulus package in history by the American Congress. For example, Novartis increased its lobbying expenditures by 259% and Biogen by 344%. The authors argue that the return on investment on a dollar of lobbying is much higher than a dollar of R&D.

The most controversial – and often unspoken – influence of Big Pharma is the existence of automated trade deals between pharmaceutical companies and governments. The WHO announcement of a pandemic automatically triggered advance-purchase agreements with pharmaceutical companies for millions of doses of a pandemic influenza vaccine (Lakoff, 2017). The UK and USA currently have contracts with six pharmaceutical companies, guaranteeing that they will be served first before other countries, with strict patent protection agreements, leading to criticism over international solidarity (*Financial Times*, 18/07/2020). Pharmaceutical companies also have an agreement that they are not legally liable for any side effects or deaths from any COVID-19 vaccinations, as they have had insufficient time to test the long-term effects (who.int, 10/09/2020).

Thus it seems likely that governmental decisions have been influenced to some extent by individuals with ties to Big Pharma, but the crucial question is how large and how decisive this influence has been. In the complex reality of incremental governmental decision-making processes, it seems difficult to give a conclusive answer.

INTERNATIONAL INSTITUTIONS

World Health Organisation: A key political player during this pandemic is the WHO, which is 'the United Nations specialised agency for public health, providing technical cooperation, carrying out programmes to control and eradicate disease and striving to improve the quality of human life', with 'a core responsibility in the area of research and coordination of research' (who.int).

In December 2019, when a cluster of pneumonia cases was discovered in Wuhan, the WHO immediately activated their emergency management team. They released their first package of guidance on 10 January 2020. Several days later, their R&D Blueprint for preventing epidemics was activated; this Blueprint had been approved in 2016 by the 194 WHO member states to accelerate research and development during an epidemic.

The WHO had developed this plan in response to their failure to quickly provide vaccines, treatments, diagnostics, and medical teams during the Ebola outbreak in West Africa in 2014. Critical reports about the Ebola outbreak had identified several bottlenecks, including a lack of funding and transparency. The Ebola experience had also taught them that it is possible to compress R&D timelines from a decade or longer to less than a single year if there is the international will and funding and more global coordination of national and regional R&D initiatives by the WHO. This blueprint offers technical guidance, coordination (e.g. avoiding unnecessary duplication, addressing priorities) and the outlining of funding processes, appropriate incentives, and other measures. On 11–12 February 2020, the WHO convened the Global Research Forum, bringing researchers and funders together, to stimulate and coordinate R&D. The WHO collected almost a billion from states and private donor, including from pharmaceutical giants.

The WHO Emergency Committee coordinates the response to COVID-19, and works together with the Global Outbreak Alert and Response Network (GOARN) which is 'a collaboration of institutions and networks that pools human and technical resources for rapid identification, confirmation and response to outbreaks of international importance, including the COVID-19 outbreak'. This network includes, among others, universities, research institutes, commercial laboratories and pharmaceutical companies. The actions from the Emergency Committee and GOARN helped to fast-track the development of diagnostics, therapeutics, and vaccines.

On 30 January, the WHO announced the highest level of international alert and on 11 March a pandemic was declared (who.int). The WHO used these announcements as early as February to call countries to start prevention and control, buy PPE and medical equipment, and 'test-test-test' to get data about the spread of the pandemic. Based on the latest research, the WHO has been advising to maintain a physical distance between people, to wash hands frequently, and to give medical masks to specific groups and non-medical masks to the general public when physical distancing is not possible, for example on public transport.

However, the dedication of all resources into finding the pandemic Holy Grail, a vaccine, has been criticised by experts, as the virus may have mutated by the time that a vaccine becomes available, as animals can also spread this zoonotic virus. However, we will not vaccinate animals, and developing a vaccine is extremely expensive and time-consuming as it has a failure rate of 90% (Gouglas et al., 2018). Even though politicians claim that the vaccines will stop the pandemic, the clinical trials do not look at outcomes such as a reduction in long hospital admissions, use of Intensive Care Units, mortality rates, or the interruption of transmission of the virus (Doshi, 2020). Ongoing Phase III trials seem to focus on the reduction of any mild symptoms as the primary outcome measure, which means that if a trial participant coughs less frequently than before the trial they may already help the vaccine trial coming closer to its successful completion. Trials also seem to focus dominantly on healthy people and do not seem to include enough individuals from vulnerable subgroups who suffer disproportionally from COVID-19, such as elderly people or minorities (ibidem). Furthermore, it is uncertain whether the vaccine will be effective as the virus may have mutated by the time that is released. Furthermore, in general, there is little uptake of vaccinations, even during epidemics (Bish et al., 2011); therefore, the British minister of health is considering making vaccinations compulsory for the entire population, even though scientists strongly object to such an authoritarian step (*Guardian*, 29/09/2020). However, even though the trials are still far from completed, the UK has already bought 340 million doses of vaccinations, worth most likely several billions; the question is how likely it is when so much money is at stake that the approving medical bodies could make an independent judgement, including the option of rejection of the findings from these trials (Torjeson, 2020). For reasons like these, some journalists have wondered whether the governmental mantras about vaccinations as the ultimate elixir, ending all our suffering, may be more symbolic than realistic.

Private-public partnerships: At the start of the 20th century, John Rockefeller argued that the best approach to combating poverty was less regulation and more philanthropy (McGoey, 2015), as Matthew Bishop and Michael Green wrote in their book *Philanthrocapitalism* (2010): 'the rich can get shit done'. As Rockefeller's three-year-old grandson had died from scarlet fever, Rockefeller invested heavily in biomedical research, which seemed to stimulate other philanthropists to focus on biomedical science as well. Philanthrocapitalism seems to bring a capitalist way of problem-solving to global healthcare and often includes the idea that philanthropy and profit-making can go hand-in-hand. It seems that these private-public partnerships give a larger role to pharmaceutical companies, such as Gavi, the Vaccine Alliance, which has reserved seats for vaccine companies whose primary income comes from Gavi. This conflict of interests has led to significant criticism, as these companies may influence priority-setting and fund-allocation (Clinton & Sridhar, 2017). Similar to the WHO, Gavi has invested in developing vaccines, and the Bill and Melinda Gates Foundation has promised to sponsor up to 100 million doses of COVID-19 vaccines for low- and middle-income countries.

Vertical approach: Although philanthropy by capitalists seems to have helped to limit or eradicate some global diseases, there is no evidence that it has reduced poverty or socio-economic inequality (McGoey, 2015). The main reason for this is that philanthropists seem to prefer a so-called vertical approach: they focus on specific (infectious) diseases and their eradication, as their effectiveness can easily be quantified and measured (Clinton & Sridhar, 2017). A good example is Gavi, which was initiated by the Bill and Melinda Gates Foundation.

However, both philanthropists and nations have invested relatively little in basic healthcare infrastructures and socio-economic equality which seem crucial for global health (ibid.). Consequently, when an epidemic happens in an underdeveloped region, people may lack the structural healthcare resources for an efficient response, and the epidemic can quickly escalate to a pandemic. Research suggests that pandemics such as COVID-19 and SARS have an unequal impact on individuals with low socio-economic status and on developing regions (see Chapter 3). Thus, medical philanthropy seems like gig-giving and not structural development. In contrast with this trend of vertical philanthropy, research suggests that basic health-care systems can create a more efficient response to a pandemic and decrease the severity of diseases (ibid.). Several reasons for this vertical approach have been suggested, from the selfish (a philanthropist may like the idea that they have eradicated one specific disease) to ensuring that healthcare systems remain so bad that pandemics can run their course and pharmaceutical companies can continue selling their treatments and vaccinations during epidemics. A logical conclusion would be that the COVID-19 may not have escalated as much as it has, and at least it would not have had such an unequal impact if international health organisations had had a more horizontal approach to global health.

Criticisms: Many of the international health organisations, including the WHO, Gavi, the World Trade Organisation, and the World Bank, lack political power; they cannot, for example, demand financial contributions or sanction countries. Contributions are often voluntary, and funds for pandemics are raised ad hoc, such as the big donor conference for COVID-19 in February 2020. This lack of political power could make international health organisations vulnerable to demands from donors as to how the money gets spent (Godlee, 1994). For example, the WHO has received much criticism regarding its lack of financial transparency and the influences from its sponsors (Clinton & Sridhar, 2017); it seems that they have listened to this criticism, as during the COVID-19 pandemic they have been publishing detailed budgets. The WHO has also been criticised for having to buy in outside external expertise which they do not have in-house; this could make their decision-making more vulnerable to commercial interests (ibid.). However, the R&D Blueprint created more clarity about agent monitoring, and during COVID-19 there seems to be clearer independence of the roles of WHO decision-makers.

In the past, the WHO Emergency Committee has been criticised for hiding its decisions from public scrutiny, but during COVID-19, proceedings of their meetings have been made available online. However, no proceedings can be found about the decision-making process to declare COVID-19 a pandemic, with only general data trends reported in the press conference and no overview of data and research which led to this decision. This lack of transparency is surprising, given that this announcement triggered international and national mechanisms, including automatic trade deals for billions of vaccines between states and pharmaceutical companies.

Let us try to reconstruct their decision to announce the pandemic. Similar to previous pandemics, the WHO was possibly facing uncertain data of a new virus which could potentially lead to many deaths, and – in contrast to their late and small response to the Ebola outbreak – they seem to have decided this time to be 'better safe than sorry' (Bjørkdahl & Carlsen, 2019; Lakoff, 2017). It has been argued that they seem to be doing everything to avoid that they may be negatively judged in future 'Corona Nuremberg Trials' for having contributed to preventable deaths – like during the Ebola pandemic; thus, it has been argued that their actions are more led by their fear of losing face and power than by scientific data (Levy, 2020). As French President Sarkozy said during a previous pandemic: 'I will always prefer to be too prudent than not enough' (Lakoff, 2017, p.109). Furthermore, in 2010 the WHO had removed the criterion of the disease severity to identify a pandemic; this meant that the number of deaths is not relevant to calling something a pandemic, as some studies suggest that the mortality rates of COVID-19 are only slightly larger than seasonal flu (Lakoff, 2017). This meant that a relatively mild pandemic could trigger a strong response from the WHO.

WHO Communication: Researchers have estimated that approximately 800 people have died globally due to so-called 'misinformation' about COVID-19, which confirms similar trends during previous pandemics (Bjørkdahl & Carlsen,

2019; Islam et al., 2020). Thus, it is no surprise that in contrast with previous pandemics the WHO has focused much on getting the communication right. For example, a special team tackles the infodemics for the public. This WHO Information Network for Epidemics (EPI-WIN) team selects research information and communicates this in simplified and tailored forms.

In April 2020, EPI-WIN invited experts world-wide to develop a strategy on how to 'tackle the infodemics' and to 'simplify the information', which led to the publication of their report entitled 'managing the COVID-19 infodemic'. This report recommended governments to clearly communicate the threat of the virus and the need for citizens to follow easy well-described precautionary measures. The report describes for example how scientific uncertainties and critical opinions on social media could undermine the effectiveness of public health communication by 'playing down the disease threat'. Without explicating, it almost feels as if EPI-WIN wants governments to diminish the communication of scientific uncertainties, mute dissident voices, and sufficiently frighten citizens, with the aim of creating adherence to precautionary measures and manufacturing public consent for governmental health policies (cf. Bjørkdahl & Carlsen 2019).

One implementation of the EPI-WIN policy is the international awareness campaign started by the British government about the risks of incorrect and false information regarding the pandemic: 'Stop the Spread'. Furthermore, several countries have also set up groups of experts on communication and behaviour, such as the British Scientific Pandemic Influenza group on Behaviour and Communications (SPI-B&C). The publicly available advisory documents from the latter committee were unfortunately surprisingly brief and included limited research findings on risk-perception and mental health, as described in this book. Their main recommendations focused on keeping government communication as clear and simple as possible, to create public consent for national health policies and to stimulate adherence to public health guidelines. These minutes almost read like recommendations to control citizen behaviour without paying attention to the psychological black-box of subjective experiences, perceptions and motivations behind individual actions (Vos, 2011). The next chapters in this book will open this psychological black-box.

PREPAREDNESS

Many epidemiologists and virologists foresaw the emergence of a pandemic. For example, the failed response to Ebola led to the conclusion by many organisations that this 'was a stark reminder of the fragility of health security in an interdependent world, and of the importance of building a more robust global system so that all people may be protected from such threats' (Clinton & Sridhar, 2017, p.3). In their 2016 R&D Blueprint, the WHO identified coronaviruses – such as SARS – as a particular potential threat. The Annual Meeting of the World Economic Forum in Davos had concluded in January 2016 that the world is at risk of pandemics. Therefore they started the Coalition for Epidemic Preparedness Innovation (CEPI), where stakeholders from governments, foundations, industry, and civil society discussed the urgent need for a fresh approach to pandemics. On 12 February 2018, the WHO Director-General Ghebreyesus warned at the World Government Summit that a devastating epidemic could emerge and kill millions of people because of a lack of preparation. These experts could foresee this pandemic as they were aware of the structural lack of preparedness, and the significant risks posed by global ecological collapse and living in a hyper-connected world (as will be described in the next chapter).

Led by these experts, politicians stepped up, including US President Barack Obama, who had written a letter to a newspaper in 2015 saying that nations should prepare themselves for future pandemics. For example, American authorities conducted a number of exercises, though mostly focused on large-scale pandemics of a virus with large infection and mortality rates, usually in the context of bioterrorism (Lakoff, 2017). These exercises led to the develop-ment of national guidelines on how to act during extreme crisis. Consequently, civil servants seemed unprepared for a virus with moderate infection rates, low mortality rates and most likely not resulting from bio-war but originating in bats. It has been argued that governments have invested more in precaution – preventing catastrophes – and not in preparedness – knowing what to do in case of a potential emergency, including communicating to the audience that they may be wrong (ibid.). Therefore, researchers have concluded that coun-tries often 'confuse the logic of preparedness with that of precaution, and not to have considered the transformation this new logic requires in its communi-cation with the public' (Kelly et al., 2019; Sandman, 1993).

Consequently, there are 14,000 scientific articles about pandemic prepared-ness, and reading a random selection of these seems to suggest a structural lack of preparedness in many countries, which includes a lack of national coordina-tion and communication plans, availability of personal protective equipment, sufficient medical equipment such as ventilators, and risks to staffing. For exam-ple, the UK's biological security strategy was published in 2018 to address the threat of pandemics. However, this strategy was not properly implemented, according to a former government chief scientific advisor. Professor Sir Ian Boyd blamed this on a lack of resources; his statement was supported by other civil servants who described a political unwillingness to invest in pandemic preparedness. Furthermore, the NHS failed a government test of its ability to handle a pandemic, Exercise Cygnus, in October 2016. This exercise showed that the pandemic would cause the country's health system to collapse from a lack of resources, mainly due to a lack of ventilators, PPE and the logistics of the disposal of dead bodies. However, the details of this report remain classified. Similar conclusions seem to apply to the 2019 'Influenza Preparedness Strategy', which considers seasonal influenza outbreaks. These strategy reports include many recommendations, such as developing coordination and communication plans and purchasing sufficient face-masks and respirators; they described these preparations as of high national urgency. A 2019 parliamentary inquiry into biological security was postponed and then cancelled because MPs regarded this as less important than other priorities (Carrington, 2020; Nuki & Gardner, 2020; Pegg, 2020).

'We were utterly unprepared. Our managers brushed off the dust from our pandemic plans, but we did not know what this was really about; we were improvising. We are masters in improvisation, but you cannot improvise with zero resources, while the management is pressuring us not to improvise and instead stick to the rules – which rules? There are no rules! We knew that we only had PPE for one or two months, and we knew that the number of ventilators would quickly become insufficient at the ICU. However, our hospital struggled to buy the PPE and ventilators we needed, as all purchases had to go via formal, slow procurement, and the government refused to buy PPE and ventilators on a large scale. We made our own garments from binbags – imagine being a patient and seeing nurses in binbags! However, in the end the peak that we feared that would happen, has never happened; yes we were unprepared for the small peak that happened, but – thank God – we have not seen the worst-case scenario that the government was warning us for. At one point, the government seemed to have become so afraid for the worst-case scenario, that they shut down all other departments in the hospital 'to free up resources', they said. Whereas they initially overestimated our ability to cope with a little spike in the number of patients – due to years of under-preparing and under-funding – later they underestimated our ability by freeing up too many resources. Consequently, most nurses and doctors have been doing nothing for many months. The people are clapping for us, each Thursday night, but most of us are simply sitting at home, doing nothing. This government has failed, first by not preparing us for the pandemic, and second when it happened they played panic-football. Many patients have died unnecessarily – initially due to a lack of equipment, and later due to the closure of other departments, such as life-saving oncology check-ups.'
(Interviewee Emma)

UNCERTAIN DATA

'We have a simple message for all countries: test, test, test.' These are the famous words of WHO Director General Dr Tedros Adhanom Ghebreyesus in the media briefing on COVID-19 on 16 March 2020. His mantra quickly went viral in the press and the social media: 'Test, test, test—that is the credo at the moment, and it is the only way to really understand how much the coronavirus is spreading.' If testing is the credo, then the belief in the test must be very strong, lifting it to almost a religious status. However, already in 2007, Gina Kolata warned in the *New York Times* of the wrong use of tests and paradigmatic faith in tests: '*Faith in Quick Test Leads to Epidemic That Wasn't*' (22/01/2007). How strong is the scientific evidence for the reliability of the tests? How useful are the tests? We have already heard the story of Martin about the uncertainty of data in his health trust. He is not the only person pointing at the uncertainty of data, as there seem to be five fundamental problems with data collection – even though public health announcements often seem to create the image that scientists can precisely explain what is going on and that politicians can control the pandemic.

First problem: The first problem is that the tests may not be completely reliable. As this so-called 'novel coronavirus' is indeed still novel, and COVID-19 is a new disease, there seems to be insufficient information about the tests. The American Center for Disease Control (CDC) has reported that depending on the test, up to 50% of the diagnoses might be wrong (CDC, 23/05/2020). For example, molecular tests – also called PCR tests, viral RNA tests or nucleic acid tests – look for genetic material that may potentially come from the virus. The PCR test does this by selecting an area of the DNA where the virus is expected to be and subsequently this area is many times amplified to make it easily detectable. However, this means that the researchers select the target area beforehand and do not amplify other areas, even though it may be possible that the virus is bound to another, unselected area which is still unknown to researchers. Formulated more formally: the PCR tests are calibrated for the specific RNA-sequences which are assumed to be associated with SARS-CoV-2, but SARS-CoV-2 does not seem to have been isolated and purified to the highest scientific standards (Watson et al., 2020). The problem seems to be that there is no gold standard to compare the test results with, like the sensitivity and specificity of a pregnancy test can be determined by examining whether the woman bears a child or not; however, for the coronavirus which does not always present itself in clear symptoms, there is not such a clear gold standard (Watson et al., 2020).

On the on one hand, due to these problems new mutations of the virus may be less likely to be detected by PCR tests, and many studies indicate a large likelihood of false-negatives, that is the lack of detecting the virus in the sample even though the patient has all the symptoms. The amplification technique also means that any tiny deviations or contaminations in the target area will be enlarged, which creates misleading or ambiguous results. Therefore, on the other hand, several studies indicate a large likelihood of false-positive test results, which means that the test tells that there is a virus even though there is not actually a virus present. Furthermore, the findings from PCR tests are rarely replicated in live culture studies, in which patient tissue samples are used to grow cultures in the laboratory, which may be a more reliable but more expensive and time-consuming test (Jefferson et al., 2020).

In sum, PCR tests have been criticised for the large number of false-positives and false-negatives, and a lack of a gold standard (Cohen et al., 2020; Surkova et al., 2020). Even the leading Centre for Disease Control wrote in their report 'CDC 2019-Novel Coronavirus (2019-nCoV) Real-Time RT-PCR Diagnostic Panel' that 'detection of viral RNA may not indicate the presence of infectious virus or that 2019-nCoV is the causative agent for clinical symptoms. (…) This test cannot rule out diseases caused by other bacterial or viral pathogens.' The instruction manuals of several PCR tests, as for instance in those by Altona Diagnostics Creative Diagnostics and Roche, state that 'these assays are not intended for use as an aid in the diagnosis of coronavirus infection' (Engelbrecht & Demeter in *The Offguardian*, 27/06/2020).

Furthermore, on 26th November 2020, a consortium of scientists have requested the retraction of an article by Corman & Drosten which has been promoted by the WHO as a blueprint to justify the use of PCR tests to detect SARS-CoV-2; the authors argued that this article is full of fundamental flaws, such as low quality of designs and protocols, extremely large number of amplification cycles (with amplification cycles more than 35, the probability that a person is actually infected is less than 3%), a possible lack of peer review and possible unreported serious conflicts of interest of Corman and Drosten (Borger et al on cormandrostenreview.com).

The alternative antigen test identifies protein fragments from the virus which offers test results in minutes; the American Food and Drug Administration does not recommend this test as false test results can be as high as 50% (FDA, 12/08/2020). For example, there is also insufficient evidence for the effectiveness of screening travellers with such tests when they enter or leave a country – for example at airports – as almost half of all test results seem inaccurate (Chetty et al., 2020). Antibody tests check for antibodies that the body's immune system has produced in response to an infection in the past; however, this test needs to be conducted in a small time frame after the symptoms of the virus emerged, and thus this test is also associated with up to 30% of false test results (*Science*, 22/05/2020).

In sum, it is not clear exactly how accurate any test is, and accuracies seem to differ per interpretation method and per laboratory (Engelbrecht & Demeter in *The Offguardian*, 27/06/2020). Population-wide screening will most likely give a false sense of certainty, while some infected people will be missed and healthy individuals may be inaccurately diagnosed (Iacobucci, 2020).

Second problem: The second problem in the data collection is the lack of a consistent and comprehensive system to record COVID-19 test results across countries and within countries. In several countries, such as the USA and the UK, the cause of deaths in care homes has not been recorded, at least during the start of the pandemic, which may underestimate figures (Betrus, 2020). The British government has also refused to publish the number of NHS staff who died from COVID-19, although independent researchers suggest that this could be around 650 (*The Independent*, 17/08/2020).

Furthermore, in response to criticisms about the specificity and sensitivity of the PCR and antigen tests to detect Sars-CoV-2, several governments have decided to determine the infection rates on the basis of the number of patients who show any COVID-19 symptoms. However, this led to many false-positive test results, as the symptoms may not have been caused by COVID-19, for example due to the seasonal flu. Consequently, while in several countries the numbers of patients identified with seasonal flu decreased significantly, the number of COVID-19 diagnoses increased – which suggests a wrong diagnosis and overestimation of COVID-19 infections. Several pathologists have also told the press how guidance on autopsies was changed early on in the pandemic, as they were asked to attribute a death to COVID-19 if the patient had any symptoms and/or if they lived together with other patients with positive test results. These pathologists argue that it is impossible to say who has died from COVID-19, who has died from another disease but happened to have a positive COVID-19 test, and who has died from another disease but were suspected of some COVID-19 symptoms without a positive test result (e.g. *The Spectator*, 30/05/2020; *Tubantia*, 23/05/2020; *RTV News*, 28/05/2020). Due to the criticisms to using symptoms to diagnose COVID-19, the British Department of Health and Social Care had to lower the total number of COVID-19-related deaths by 12.5% (*The Guardian*, 13/08/2020).

Third problem: The third problem is how the collected data is interpreted and compared with other diseases and compared across countries. Several authors have argued that Sars-Cov-2 has a slightly higher transmission rate than seasonal flu. The mortality rate of hospitalised patients with a COVID-19 diagnosis also seems similar or slightly higher compared to seasonal influenza (about 6%; Pormohammed et al., 2020; Wu et al., 2020). A systematic review of studies on the lethality of COVID-19 also suggests similar risks as seasonal flu (Swiss Policy Research Institute, 24/10/2020).

However, it seems dangerous to generalise findings, as these studies also suggest that certain countries and regions have larger infection and mortality rates than others and that the health-care systems are better prepared in certain countries and regions than others (Noor & Islam, 2020). The pandemic also seems to have a different impact on individuals with comorbid physical diseases, such as cardiovascular diseases, reduced immune system functioning or obesity; they seem to have larger likelihoods of infection, severe symptoms, and mortality (Kim et al., 2020; Luo et al., 2020). Certain lifestyles, such as smoking and alcohol use, also seem to increase infection and mortality rates (Abate et al., 2020). This variation may not only be caused by different mutations of the virus, but the infection and mortality rates may also be influenced by other factors, such as ethnicity and socio-economic inequality (see next chapter). Another problem is that up to one-third of all hospitalised individuals with COVID-19 symptoms will continue experiencing symptoms in the long term, which can have a large impact on the health-care system (Rimmer, 2020). Thus there are large variations in the impact of the virus, and it seems difficult to make generalised statements about how the pandemic behaves in each region and for each population. Some researchers have also argued that public health policies should focus on supporting the weakest link – the hotspot regions and the most vulnerable population groups – instead of trusting the average impact, like stopping one leak in a dyke along a river to prevent the rest of the dyke falling apart at a later stage.

Fourth problem: The fourth problem is that describing the number of excess deaths may also not reveal the direct impact of COVID-19. That is, because the tests and data collection do not seem to be completely reliable, some government agencies have decided to focus on the number of extra deaths in 2020 compared to the same period in previous years, without looking at the reason of why more people died. These researchers seem to assume that the extra deaths can be largely attributed to the COVID-19 virus. However, several British institutes have reported that many excess deaths are due to the lockdown, as for example many hospital departments have been closed and patients have missed out on health checks and surgeries (DHSC, ONS, GAD & HO, 2020).

Fifth problem: The fifth problem is that the companies responsible for the track-and-trace system may not have been delivering what they promised. This system involves individuals leaving their contact details for every public place they go, so that they can be warned via phone or email if they have been near an infected person. The expectations of this system were high, as a mathematical study from Imperial College found if test and trace worked quickly and effectively, the R number could potentially be reduced by up to 26%. However, similar to the problems with Ferguson's calculations – as we will see below – these colleagues also seemed to ignore the psychological and social realities of the track-and-trace system.

For example, the British government has been overestimating the number of conducted tests by almost 75% (*Sky News*, 12/07/2020; *The Guardian*, 13/10/2020). Only one quarter of the actual cases seemed to be picked up by the test and trace system during 2020 (House of Commons, Science and Technology Committee, 17/09/2020). One of the problems is that only 74% of all individuals in the contact-tracing systems were reached, and that even one quarter of those who were asked to go for a test in one of the 500 local testing centres were turned away due to a lack of capacity (*The Guardian*, 13/10/2020). More than 16,000 potentially infected individuals were also not contacted due to an avoidable failure, as the track-and-trace system runs on Excel, and the Excel database had run out of columns to register these individuals (*Metro*, 5/10/2020).

It has been argued that these failures are caused by the fact that the track-and-trace system was not run locally, but centrally, as experience suggests that local systems are more effective (Mahase, 2020a). The contracts for creating this £12 billion centralised system were handed to the private companies Deloitte and Serco and their subcontractors, who had limited experience with setting up such systems. This work is also overseen by a committee with members such as the chairperson Dido Harding who have limited, no or even negative track records with setting up such systems; the committee only includes one public health expert (*Local Government Chronicle*, 15/09/2020). Several journalists have described how the companies who received the contracts and the individuals on the panel all seemed to have close personal or financial connections to the government or the conservative party; therefore, one British columnist concluded: 'the test-and-trace system might be a public health fiasco, but it's a private profit bonanza. Consultants at one of the companies involved have each been earning £6,000 a day. Massive contracts have been awarded without competitive tendering. Astonishingly, at least one of these, worth £410m and issued to Serco, contains no penalty clause: even if Serco fails to fulfil its terms, it gets paid in full.' (Monbiot in *The Guardian*, 21/10/2020)

In addition to the suspected nepotism in the allocation of contracts, there is a more fundamental question of whether any track-and-trace system would ever function perfectly. The estimated effects of the track-and-trace system assume that at least 80% of a case's contacts will isolate themselves (SAGE minutes, 1/05/2020). However, in reality, less than 20% of them fully self-isolate, particularly the youngest and the poorest individuals (SPI minutes, 16/09/2020). This seems to confirm other studies, which show that only 18% of people with symptoms stayed at home, particularly due to the financial implications (Atchison et al., 2020). Only privileged people may be able to afford staying at home for self-isolation.

THE NUDGING PARADIGM

In sum, there are many uncertainties about the adequacy of the tests and their interpretations, about the track-and-trace system and about the independence of scientific advisors in general. How is it possible that despite these uncertainties, governments have decided on drastic measures such as nationwide lockdowns? Which psychological and social processes happened when uncertain science was translated into certain governmental policies?

In response to questions like these, several independent groups of researchers have launched their own independent advisory committees on COVID-19 – such as the British independent Sage Group. They have been joined by other journalists and scientists expressing their scepticism about the continuously repeated numbers of COVID-19 deaths in the daily press briefings in the White House and 10 Downing Street, and about the unfounded health policies that were based on these uncertain figures (German Network for Evidence-Based Medicine, 20/03/2020; Ioannidis, 2020a, 2020b, 2020c; Ioannidis et al., 2020, Levit, 2020; Roussell, in *OffGuardian*, 24/03/2020). They have argued that the infection and mortality rates do not seem to warrant the large-scale panic and nationwide lockdowns.

Some critical authors have also argued, that the data have deliberately been manipulated (Reiss & Bakhdi, 2020). For example, an email leaked to Danish *newspaper Politiken* has indicated that some Danish politicians may have pressured scientists to deliberately overstate the danger (*Politiken*, 28/05/2020, 29/05/2020). In the UK, several anonymous sources have reported that the top advisor of the Prime Minister, Dominic Cummings, had been pushing scientists to exaggerate the severity of COVID-19, to support a nationwide lockdown (Bloomberg, 28/04/2020). Furthermore, a leaked – and later contested – document that allegedly contains minutes from the German Corona taskforce described that the German government wanted to increase the public sense of threat of the pandemic – for example by exaggerating the infection and mortality data. This document suggests that focusing the public health communication on the existential threat may increase the likelihood that citizens follow the governmental guidelines.

Why have these individual governmental officials pressured scientists? Some journalists have suggested that these politicians may have been pressured themselves by lobbyists of Big Pharma or Big Tech, to give higher mortality rates to justify investments in medical equipment and vaccinations. The pressure could also be the result of cognitive dissonance reduction, or more simply said: preventing loss of face, as the governments had already decided for a lockdown and they did not like any data suggesting that the lockdown may have been unnecessary.

Some sceptical authors have also argued that the repetition of exaggerated numbers in the daily press meetings created the sense of existential threat, which could stimulate a less critical attitude of citizens towards their government: 'a reliable way to make people believe in falsehoods is frequent repetition, because familiarity is not easily distinguished from truth; authoritarian institutions and marketers have always known this fact' (Kahneman, 2016, p.87). This focus on threats in the public health communication seems to follow from the recommendations from the WHO Information Network for Epidemics. As such, this is also nothing new, as traditional handbooks and guidelines on public health communication often seem to recommend this type of existential communication (Guttmann, 2000; Sellnow et al., 2008).

This includes for example the book 'Nudge' which suggests that 'a choice architect has the responsibility for organising the context in which people make decisions' (Thaler & Sunstein, 2009, p.36). Several political leaders who are currently in power seemed to have explicitly used nudging in their political campaigns or during their administration, such as the scandal of manipulating Brexit-voters by Cambridge Analytica (Vos, 2020). The nudge paradigm has also explicitly been used by possibly the most influential British companies during the pandemic: the Behavioural Insights Team (BIT), nicknamed 'the nudge unit'. Furthermore, the main advisor of the British Prime Minister, Dominic Cummings, came into the public spotlight for his advisory role on nudging undecided voters during the Brexit campaign, and he seems to have recommended similar nudging strategies during this pandemic (Bloomberg, 28/04/2020). Thus, governmental advisors seem to have been blindly following the traditional scientific paradigm of psychologically nudging the population into obedience via repeatedly communicating existential threats (even though the science behind the effectiveness of existential nudging is very thin, as we will see in later chapters).

Thus, epidemiological facts – 'the First Pandemic' – do not seem to explain the strong public and governmental responses to the pandemic on their own. To explain these responses, we need first and foremost to understand the 'Second Pandemic' of political decision-making and psychological processes.

Should we therefore also conclude that the pandemic is nothing else than mind manipulation and lobbying? No. Some criticasters seem to make an induction fallacy in their reasoning. Their conclusion that the pandemic is totally fake seems to be an overgeneralisation of their observation that political and psychological processes have shaped the pandemic, and that some individuals have used the opportunities of the pandemic for their own benefit. As argued in this chapter, there is indeed strong evidence for powerful individuals and companies influencing the governmental responses to the pandemic, and governments seem to have just been muddling through instead of making the most evidence-based decisions. I call these 'conspiracies' with a small letter to describe these small influences during the incremental governmental decision-making processes. However, there seems less evidence for 'One Big Conspiracy' with capital letters, suggesting that the pandemic was deliberately created and spread – or that there is no pandemic at all – to control the population or to increase commercial profits.

Researchers on the psychology of conspiracy theories often use the rule-of-thumb that the more people are involved in a conspiracy, the less likely the conspiracy is to be true, because it is more likely that there will be some whistle-blowers amongst a large group of conspiricists (Uscinski et al., 2020). A more likely hypothesis seems to be that governmental responses to the pandemic seem to be the result of a desire of politicians to look in-control and in-the-know – even despite the reality of scientific uncertainties, organisational incompetence, institutional muddling-through, opportunities for lobbyists and nepotism, and governmental unwillingness to prepare for large-scale pandemics. The following two sections will exemplify how such social and psychological processes played a role when the British government translated scientific uncertainties into public health policies.

HERD IMMUNITY

On the one hand, when countries identified the first COVID-19 cases, countries such as China, Italy and France followed the WHO pandemic guidelines and played safe by enforcing strict regional or nationwide lockdowns.

On the other hand, countries including the UK and the USA postponed a lockdown and large-scale preparations, including rejecting the calls from scientific advisory committees to buy PPE and ventilators (UK House of Lords COVID Committee, July 2020). Instead, a day after the WHO announced the pandemic, on 12 March, the British PM Boris Johnson announced in the daily press conference that the government would no longer try to track and trace the contacts of every suspected case, and instead they offered soft advice – i.e. people with symptoms should stay at home. This strategy was aimed at delaying the pandemic, although this could mean that 'many people should expect to lose loved ones' according to the PM. Sir Patrick Vallance, the UK's chief scientific advisor, explained this further on Sky News (12/03/2020): the UK would suppress the virus but not get rid of it entirely while focusing on protecting vulnerable groups. In the meantime, up to 60% of the population could get sick, but as the virus causes milder illness in younger age groups, most would recover and subsequently be immune to the virus. This 'herd immunity' would reduce the transmission and resurgence of the virus. However, Johnson faced much criticism from the public and medical scientists. Several experts argued that there were still many uncertain factors regarding the basic data and the virus in general, including uncertainties about the building of antibodies and about becoming immune to a second infection. This meant that there was a significant risk that herd immunity would not work, and in these times of uncertainty, these experts wanted to play it safe.

Meanwhile, Prime Minister Johnson also referred to a piece of advice from the Behavioural Insights Team (BIT) that a lockdown early during the pandemic could lead to 'behavioural fatigue': if restrictions come into force too early, people could become increasingly uncooperative and less vigilant, before the peak of the pandemic had even started. However, there is no clear definition of what behavioural fatigue is, there is no research on this, and the idea seems to have been made-up by one of the BIT-advisors (Mahase, 2020b). On 16 March, 681 behavioural scientists signed an open letter to the government raising concerns over the evidence behind this concept: 'We are not convinced that enough is known about "behavioural fatigue" or to what extent these insights apply to the current exceptional circumstances. Such evidence is necessary if we are to base a high-risk public health strategy on it.' They added that focusing on this idea seemed to have led the government to 'believe that halting the spread of the disease is impossible'.

QUARANTINE

The discussion about herd immunity reminds us of Esposito's concept of social immunisation (2011), as we will see in the next chapter: the idea that life needs to be protected from itself and needs, therefore, to be exposed to death. The psychological pseudo-concept of behavioural fatigue seemed to be invented as a biopolitical mechanism, speaking in dehumanised terms about flocks – the deaths of loved ones may not sound so bad when compared with the deaths of animals – and a wise, protective shepherd. Individuals are reduced to bare life, stripped of their meaningfulness (Agamben, 2020a, 2020b). This is thanato politics at its worst: politicians decide who can be sacrificed – such as individuals with low socio-economic status and ethnic minorities, as government studies had already shown that COVID-19 affects these groups more than others. The next chapter will elaborate these ideas.

This political approach has been described elsewhere as 'functionalism': we reduce individuals to a mere variable in a statistical function (Vos, 2020), such as the SIR-model: Total population N = Susceptible S + Infected I + Removed R (recovered or dead). It is this functionalistic approach that would ultimately determine the decision of the British government to have a nationwide lockdown – going against the evidence provided by the governmental advisory committee (SPI-B&C) which warned about the negative side effects of large-scale quarantine (see next chapter).

The hypothesis that an entire country could be put in lockdown was raised for the first time in 2006 in the context of eradicating smallpox. The authors Henderson and Borio (2006) concluded that a nationwide lockdown would be undesirable as this could 'result in significant disruption of the social functioning of communities and result in possibly serious economic problems'. Therefore, he argued that herd immunity is the only reasonable alternative – the lesser of two evils. In a later study, Henderson and colleagues concluded (Inglesby et al., 2006):

> 'There are no historical observations or scientific studies that support the confinement by quarantine of groups of possibly infected people for extended periods in order to slow the spread of influenza. A World Health Organization (WHO) Writing Group, after reviewing the literature and considering contemporary international experience, concluded that "forced isolation and quarantine are ineffective and impractical." Despite this recommendation by experts, mandatory large-scale quarantine continues to be considered as an option by some authorities and government officials. The interest in quarantine reflects the views and conditions prevalent more than fifty years ago, when much less was known about the epidemiology of infectious diseases and when there was far less international and domestic travel in a less densely populated world. It is difficult to identify circumstances in the past half-century when large-scale quarantine has been

effectively used in the control of any disease. The negative consequences of large-scale quarantine are so extreme (forced confinement of sick people with the well; complete restriction of movement of large populations; difficulty in getting critical supplies, medicines, and food to people inside the quarantine zone) that this mitigation measure should be eliminated from serious consideration.'

Local and regional lockdowns have been implemented before, for example in response to the SARS-pandemic in China and Canada. Yet, until recently, international health organisations such as the WHO advised against nationwide lockdowns. Existing research about local or regional lockdowns also casted doubts about the psychological and social side effects (Brooks et al., 2020). Thus, there was no history of scientific support for the idea of nationwide lockdowns. Also, China did not have a nationwide lockdown, but only shut down Wuhan and Hubei. How did we go within a couple of months from a scientific consensus against lockdown to governments putting four billion people in more than 100 countries in lockdown? How could governments convince their citizens that this was the best measure to halt the pandemic? How was it possible that governments called these lockdowns 'scientific', even though 6,500 scientists and health-care workers, supported by more than 60,000 individuals in the general public, signed the 'Great Barrington Declaration' to the American President, telling him that there is little scientific evidence for lockdowns, and that there is 'almost no correlation' between lockdown strategies and infection rates (although since its publication, several scientists have criticised these arguments, and journalists have identified some fake signatures)?

Neil Ferguson is a British epidemiologist and professor of mathematical biology. He specialises in creating mathematical models of disease outbreaks such as foot-and-mouth disease and the swine flu; however, researchers have criticised his models for often overestimating the severity of these epidemics (Betrus, 2020). In February 2020, Ferguson led the Imperial College COVID-19 Response Team who were developing mathematical models for COVID-19. It is important to realise that these models include many theoretical assumptions which were difficult to pinpoint with full certainty at the time that these models were created (Dobson, 2020). Examples include the duration of infectiousness, the probability of transmission and the rate of contact. The key statistic is $R = 1$, the threshold value at which diseases become epidemic. The problem is that it is challenging to measure R, particularly with non-systematic testing and uncertain data recording; thus, R is always an estimate with a large variation. Both the SIR-model and the non-linear R-functions are very sensitive, and a slight increase of one of the variables – for example, a small increase in the rate of infection – can lead to a large increase in the number of infected individuals.

The estimations that Ferguson and his colleagues (2020) used in their models were larger than those of most other scientists, and assumed that only 10% of all cases were being detected in China and only one in three cases coming into the UK, and consequently the new coronavirus could affect up to 60% of the UK's population in the worst-case scenario. However, these estimates were not in line with the best available natural experiment: the infection and mortality rates at cruise ships in lockdown; the data from the *Diamond Princess* show that Ferguson's assumptions were implausible (Betrus, 2020). Mass protests, such as Black Life Matters after the death of George Floyd, also did not lead to a spike in new cases as would be predicted with Ferguson's model (ibid.). Furthermore, scientists have questioned the computer model Ferguson made, and they have not been able to replicate his findings (Boland & Zolfagharifard, 2020; Richards & Boudnik, 2020).

Another problem with Ferguson's theoretical models – and crucial to the topic of this book – was the ignorance of social dynamics, risk-perception, population behaviour and the physical and mental side effects of quarantine: he seemed to ignore the influence of the second pandemic on the first pandemic (Epstein, 19/03/2020; Wells & Lurgi, 2020). In reality, individuals have most frequent contact with the same number of friends, colleagues, and acquaintances, and thus, due to the limits of their social bubble the number of individuals they could infect is also limited. Furthermore, during pandemics, individuals listen to communications from scientists, governments, and media; this shapes their risk-perception and their risk-taking or risk-avoiding behaviour. However, Ferguson assumed that 50% of households would not comply with voluntary quarantine – without any empirical evidence (Streeck, 2020). For example, in Sweden, there was no lockdown, many people seemed to stay inside their social bubbles and avoided risky situations and meeting vulnerable individuals. Overall, it seems that Sweden may have had relatively low infection and mortality rates during COVID-19, except for a short peak in mortality figures during the summer (Kamerlin & Kasson, 2020; Pierre, 2020). Furthermore, Ferguson's mathematical scenario of the lockdown did not take into account the side effects, such as prior research which indicated that quarantine can negatively affect mental and physical health and the functioning of the immune system (Brooks et al., 2020).

It seems as if the main decision-makers were thinking in black-or-white terms: we should either go for large-scale herd immunity or for a nationwide lockdown – with both extremes having relatively little empirical evidence for their effectiveness. After the herd immunity proposal seemed to have been torpedoed in the media and by the political opposition in the UK and the US, these governments seemed keen to choose the other extreme: a nationwide lockdown. Ferguson's model seems to have come at the right time for the British and American governments when they were looking for an alternative to the controversies about herd immunity. However, in their eagerness to provide certainty to the public, they seemed to minimise or ignore the uncertainties surrounding the quarantine model, such as the errors in Ferguson's prior predictions, the lack of empirical evidence for nationwide lockdowns, and the negligence of the complex social and psychological reality in mathematical models. Ultimately, Ferguson's model led the British government to impose a strict lockdown on 23 March 2020 (Nickson et al., 2020; Singh & Adhikari, 2020) and has convinced American states to do the same – without putting sufficient measures in place to mitigate these lockdown side effects.

In contrast to the black-or-white model, several countries, including Sweden, have used a mixed approach from the beginning of the pandemic – being realistic about the uncertainties of both models – combining herd-immunity, quarantine of the most vulnerable, and discontinuing high-risk events such as large gatherings and sport or music events. The communication by health authorities as well as the public debate in Sweden seemed to focus less on splitting the world into good versus evil, and prevented the creation of the illusion that there may only be one perfect solution. The Swedish mixed model did not create the perfect solution – thousands of individuals still became infected and died – but Swedish epidemiologists such as Anders Tegnell have argued that there is no evidence that a lockdown would have lowered these numbers. At the same time, the psychological, social and economic impact seems less compared to countries with a full lockdown (BBC, 24/07/2020). A key question seems to be whether researchers and politicians only look at the short-term effects of lockdown on the number of infections and deaths due to COVID-19, or whether they also take into account the side effects of lockdown which will most likely only become visible in the long-term and not in immediate statistics (see Chapter 7). As the long-term effects are still unknown, decision-makers may be inclined to be led by short-term thinking. However, in this context of uncertainties and ambiguities, the jury is still out – and will possibly remain out, as any governmental decisions may have been imperfect. Choosing between two evils will always end up with evil, even if the lesser evil is chosen.

It is remarkable how countries with relatively socialist governmental styles, empathic communication styles, and female leaders seem to have followed a different strategy than more neoliberal governments with male leaders –

leading to fewer infections and deaths (Aldrich & Lotito, 2020; Martinez, 2020; Sergent & Stajkovic, 2020). Neoliberal governments seem to have a more functionalist and materialist approach to the world (Vos, 2020), and therefore may have been using a black-or-white approach and may have liked Ferguson's mathematical and economics-oriented model. Another factor is the lack of pandemic preparedness and the fragility of health-care systems in relatively neoliberal countries such as the UK and the USA.

Furthermore, the British advisory committee SAGE feared that the NHS was unprepared and therefore a nationwide lockdown became inevitable in their reasoning (as reflected in the governmental motto: 'Stay at Home – Protect the NHS – Save Lives'): 'The aim of a lockdown is not to stop the virus spread, but to slow it down so that hospitalizations do not exceed capacity' (Betrus, 2020). Thus, if hospitals had been prepared with larger capacity and adequate equipment, a lockdown may not have been needed; thus, the reason behind the lockdown seems to be a lack of preparedness, which is the result of consecutive governments deliberately ignoring reports about pandemic preparations. 'Meanwhile, most in the media were championing continued lockdowns without ever presenting critical data analysis. It became a circular argument: polls supported lockdowns because of the media hype, and the media hype perpetuated the lockdown argument' (Betrus, 2020, p.103).

Within two weeks of the publication of his model, Ferguson changed his forecast from 500,000 to 20,000 deaths (Betrus, 2020), and within three months he admitted that countries without a lockdown had not seen a worse pandemic trajectory (Guardian, 2/06/2020). Other governmental advisors have also admitted that they may have exaggerated their estimations and recommendations and that they may have mistrusted the population to adhere to government measures (Press Briefing, Downing Street, 6 May 2020). However, by the time that Ferguson admitted his errors, it was possibly too late for governments to admit – without losing face and voters – that its decisions had been made with inaccurate science. It is possible that the mechanisms of cognitive dissonance reduction happened at this stage, that is trying to fit the data and the research with their policies instead of fitting the policies to the data. Sadly, the consequences of the decision for a nationwide lockdown may have been considerable; it has, for example, been argued, that without a lockdown, a significant number of excess deaths due to the lockdown may have been prevented (Forbes, 23/05/2020), although the alternative could also be argued, that the lockdown may have prevented COVID-19 infections and mortality rate to spiral down (New York Times, 20/03/2020).

The World Health Organisation surprised the world by communicating on 12 October 2020 that a full lockdown should be avoided at all costs as the side effects may be too large to be ethically justifiable, although short and temporary lockdowns may be necessary in the beginning stage of a pandemic for example to prepare hospitals (*Guardian*, 12/10/2020). This advice seemed to increase the conflict between scientists and politicians; for example, in the light of the need of preparing for a second wave during the pandemic, some scientists recommended to have a temporary nationwide lockdown, but the British government rejected this recommendation by referring to the WHO statement (*Guardian*, 13/10/2020). The debate seemed black-or-white: either there is a full lockdown or there are no precautionary measures at all. Both sides of the debate seemed to transform the scientific uncertainties into certainties.

In the same week as this WHO statement, the British government introduced a tier-based system, which puts different regions into different tiers of lockdown. This seemed to do more justice to the scientific uncertainties and regional epidemiological variations. They seemed to have replaced the generic model of Ferguson by more socially realistic models of bubbles: infections do not happen with the same frequency within each social group or region. Infections seem to happen within social bubbles and may be triggered by super-spreaders; only the most affected bubbles may need to be put into a lockdown instead of the full country. However, this tier-based system does not seem to be based on scientific research, and the specific measures that should be conducted within each tier are also questioned by the government's own SAGE-advisors (*The Independent*, 15/10/2020).

HOW TO CREATE RESILIENT SCIENCE

This chapter has shown how the danse macabre between scientists and governments was based on uncertain test results, uncertain track-and-trace systems, and uncertain public health measures. The decisive scientific models and governmental decisions seem to have ignored the psychology of pandemics, such as social dynamics, risk-perception and behaviour of people. In this uncertain context, pharmaceutical lobbyists and friends of the government seem to have used the opportunities that the scientific chaos and public health urgency offered to grab a part of the financial pie.

We have also seen that possibly one of the largest causes of the escalation of the pandemic, and the need to lockdown, is the refusal of governments to prepare themselves for a range of possible future emergencies, as recommended by mountains of strategy documents dating back to years before

COVID-19. Even when governments had prepared themselves, they seemed to follow the guidelines on what to do in worst-case scenarios, and not what to do when there is a virus with a moderate infection rate and a small-to-moderate mortality rate. It seems that given this uncertain situation, wanting to avoid being responsible for many deaths and facing a Corona-Nuremberg, politicians decided for nationwide lockdowns.

To develop resilient applied science governmental advisory committees have to become independent, with members representing a wide range of relevant disciplines, and without non-expert political advisors present at meetings. Pandemic models and decision-making need to include the social and psychological reality of people. Furthermore, countries should develop strategies for a broad range of emergency scenarios and implement preparatory recommendations. Governmental and supra-governmental decision-making institutions, such as the WHO, need to be transparent, and there should be clear anti-corruption policies and accountability procedures. Pharmaceutical companies should not influence R&D priorities and strategies, and there should be sufficient non-commercial research funding. In their internal decision-making processes and external communication, health authorities should acknowledge the limitations of science and the inaccuracy of data, otherwise the general public will create false expectations of governmental policies and could start creating their own (conspiracy) theories. Above all, we may need to create more realistic expectations of science:

'Science is sometimes criticised for pretending to explain everything, for thinking that it has an answer to every question. It's a curious accusation. As every researcher working in every laboratory throughout the world knows, doing science means coming up hard against the limits of your ignorance on a daily basis – the innumerable things that you don't know and can't do. This is quite different from claiming to know everything. But if we are certain of nothing, how can we possibly rely on what science tells us? The answer is simple. Science is not reliable because it provides certainty. It is reliable because it provides us with the best answers we have at present. Science is the most we know so far about the problems confronting us. It is precisely its openness, the fact that it constantly calls current knowledge into question, which guarantees that the answers it offers are the best so far available: if you find better answers, those new answers become science. ... The answers given by science are not reliable because they are definitive. They are reliable because they are not definitive. They are reliable because they are the best answers available today. And they are the best we have because we don't consider them to be definitive, but see them as open to improvement. It's the awareness of our ignorance that gives science its reliability.' (Rovelli, 2018, p.2)

3

SOCIAL RISKS

UNCERTAIN POLITICIANS

'We animals live life in all its glorious uncertainty. Why do politicians think they can control events?' (Brown, 2009, p.10)

OVERVIEW OF THE POLITICS OF PANDEMICS

From the first moment of our Zoom conversation, I felt impressed by Carol's expertise. Behind her on my screen was a big bookcase with hundreds or possibly thousands of books. She was well-dressed, must have been in her 50s, was eloquent, spoke in professional terms, and could directly quote studies from the top of her head. Beforehand, I had read her curriculum vitae, which showed that she had published hundreds of publications on health-care management and that she sits on countless advisory boards and committees. It was her experience as an advisor during COVID-19 that I was particularly interested in. I was hoping to find some global trends in the psychology of political decision-making during COVID-19. Of course, I was aware that she works at the other side of the Atlantic, and American authorities may have different cultures, values, and histories than the United Kingdom where I work.

'Each pandemic is fundamentally political in nature,' Carol boldly stated, 'from its causes to the ways governments communicate with their citizens. To talk about pandemics is to talk about politics. As researchers we only have limited impact on political decisions: if they like our ideas they will follow us, but if they do not like our suggestions they may publicly question our authority and push through their own agenda.'

I asked Carol for an example of this.

'I have written several reports for governmental departments and other health authorities. However, several times they have decided not to do anything with my advice, and they would even not make my work available in the public domain. The problem is that I could not go public as I had signed a gagging-clause: by accepting their project, I had accepted that I could not freely speak about this. This situation has led to some difficult moral conflicts when I felt that I should speak up. Public health governance is a minefield, with many power dynamics and many uncertainties. For the average citizen, it seems difficult to know what is going on.'

This chapter will examine the psychological processes that are going on behind the political screen and the responses of individual citizens to these political processes. I will describe how politics have shaped the COVID-19 pandemic and how individual citizens feel about the pandemic and its uncertainties. Their personal experiences are embedded in this broader socio-economic-political context like the feminist movement developed the slogan 'The Personal Is Political' in the 1970s. Research shows that our general political perspective strongly determines how we perceive the pandemic and how we act, like a political filter (Allcott et al., 2020). There are, for example, significant differences between individuals in the USA who support the Republican or Democrat party: Democrats report more social distancing and see the COVID-19 risk and severity as larger than do Republicans. I will explain this from the perspective of how governments manage risks, corruption, our hyperconnected world, ecology, capitalism, biopolitics, and how powerful individuals have used the pandemic to push through their agenda.

The pinnacle of the 'ominous politization' of the pandemic is possibly the open letter that more than 1,000 current and former staff from the American Center for Disease Control wrote to the American president Trump, to ask for a greater role of their center and a smaller influence of politicians in editing or hiding their reports (*The Independent,* 18/10/2020). These individuals were preceded by the editors of the New England Journal of Medicine (6/10/2020) who for the first time in their history decided to take political sides by telling that 'dangerously incompetent politicians must go' during the upcoming US presidential election in 2020.

GOVERNMENTAL RISK MANAGEMENT MODEL

Aradau and Munster (2011) propose four different ways of how governments could respond to the uncertain situation of public risks – such as COVID-19 – which I will now describe and extend.

Table 3.1 Overview of political models, descriptions and COVID-19 examples

Political model	Description	COVID-19 examples
Governmental risk management	Governments can manage risks in multiple ways, e.g. preventing serious irreversible damage, zero-risk strategy, preventing worst-case scenario, shifting the burden of proof, preparing, declaring a state of emergency, and reducing cognitive dissonance after a policy decision.	There are examples of all governmental risk management strategies during the COVID-19 pandemic.
Corruption	Companies and powerful individuals may use the uncertainties of a pandemic for their own benefit, for example via lobbying politicians and via marketing their products.	Pharmaceutical industries have significantly invested in lobbying during the pandemic, and several companies have made large profits.
Ecology	Pandemics may be caused by human interaction with rare animal species. Due to deforestation and large-scale animal farming, there may be a larger risk for pandemics.	The SARS-CoV-2 virus seems to have originated in bats and animals in wet markets in Wuhan, China.
Hyper-connection	A virus may spread quickly between humans when there are many interactions, for example via air traffic.	The virus seems to have spread quickly due to the Chinese holiday season and to international flights.
Capitalism	The capitalist lifestyle, values and political decision-making could influence the spread and containment of a virus.	The more capitalistic characteristics a country has, the larger the infection rates and mortality rates for COVID-19.
Biopolitics	Politicians may want to control the biology of their citizens. This could imply that individual lives may need to be sacrificed for the greater good of the Life of the largest number in the population. This may be achieved via external governmental control (e.g. policing, fines) or via internal governmentality (e.g. stimulating citizens to police themselves by creating a sense of responsibility, guilt and shame).	Several governments started with external control, e.g. by imposing strict rules and policing, as reflected in the quickly approved COVID-19 emergency bills and acts. At a later stage of the pandemic, the focus shifted towards self-governmentality, where citizens are stimulated to police themselves.
State of Exception and Shock Doctrine	Politicians may call a state of emergency, and may use the shock of pandemics to push through policies which would not have been accepted in normal times.	Most countries in the world have called a state of exception, and have quickly developed and accepted emergency bills and acts which give powers to authorities which may have been unthinkable in normal times.
Inequality	Pandemics have unequal medical and socio-economic impacts in the population. Individuals with a low socio-economic status, ethnic minorities and black people are more likely to get infected and are more likely to develop severe symptoms.	COVID-19 has had large impacts on individuals with a low socio-economic status, ethnic minorities and black people. This inequality seems to have triggered civil unrest across the globe, such as the Black Lives Matter movement in the USA.

Severe irreversible damage: This is the scenario that governments want to avoid. In the face of scientific uncertainty, it is often unknown at the early stage of a pandemic whether this could progress to severe irreversible damage. By continuous monitoring of the situation, the government could estimate how likely this worst-case scenario is, and whether they should act or not. For example, the British government waited longer than in other countries before they recommended physical distancing. However, in March 2020, the COVID-19 mortality figures showed an exponential increase, followed by increasing public discontent about the lack of governmental action; this led to a tipping point for the government to impose a nationwide lockdown.

Zero-risk strategy: Governments could also apply a zero-risk strategy, whereby any risk other than zero is unjustifiable and requires intervention. Often this is the result of the public perception of risk, as it may become politically unacceptable – and imply political suicide – to take any risks. This seems to have become the strategy of European governments during COVID-19: although the mortality risks are relatively low compared to other risks – and governments do not show similar strong responses during seasonal flu – the current political narrative forced governments to enforce national lockdowns and require personal protective equipment in public spaces (see Chapter 5).

Worst-case scenario: Governments could also focus on the worst-case scenario – 'better safe than sorry'. Several authors argue that national and international health guidelines, such as the World Health Organisation (WHO), have focused on the worst-case scenarios, and thus they cannot deal proportionally to moderate risks such as COVID-19. The political actions and advice seem proportionate for a highly fatal disease such as Ebola. For example, the American government has conducted civil service exercises for bioterrorism with a coronavirus with much larger infection rates and mortality rates (Lakoff, 2017). Therefore, several health experts have recommended developing more nuanced guidelines for a range of possible future pandemics and not only the worst-case scenarios.

Shifting the burden of proof: There are multiple ways to shift the burden of proof, such as blaming 'the Chinese' or 'immigrants' for the COVID-19 pandemic. Modern governments also seem to shift the burden towards citizens (Cargile, 1997): 'you are to blame, not the government, your situation or the natural environment'. For example, governments seem to focus their communication on the lifestyles and behaviour of citizens, even though there are still many uncertainties about this and there is much more substantial evidence for the role of environmental-zoonotic factors and governments deliberately ignoring warning signs from scientists about the lack of pandemic preparedness of the health-care system.

Preparedness: Anderson (2010) has added a fifth governmental strategy. Risks can remain theoretically abstract to citizens, without any personal relevance to their physical health and life. Therefore governments need to bring the distant future to the present. Governments can, for example, do risk calculations and continuously present infection and mortality figures in daily press conferences. Governments can also imagine future risks via visioning and future planning. The WHO and other international health organisations have been leading the imagination of future risks via preparation guidelines and exercises. However, epidemiologists have complained that their preparedness plans have barely been implemented by governments (see previous chapter). The preparation often focused on having an organisation and communication plan for the worst-case scenario, but this often does not involve moderate risks with a moderate fatality, nor does it involve governments investing in material resources, such as buying sufficient personal protective equipment (PPE) and ventilators. Thus, across the board of public risks, future planning often involves recognising the structural failure of modern governments: scientists and civil servants calculate and imagine the risks, but governments only change their actual procedures slightly and allocate limited resources to risk-management (Lakoff, 2017). This has been dubbed the existential crisis of neoliberal governments (Dean, 2010).

State of emergency: When states fail due to a lack of preparedness, they may need to suddenly come up with radical action to prevent the worst-case scenario and call this a state of emergency. As will be argued below, these states of exception seem to have become the new norm, replacing politicians with long-term visions and actively preparing the country for a wide range of scenarios (Agamben, 2017, 2020b). It has, for example, been argued that many deaths, nationwide lockdowns and economic crises may have been prevented if governments had implemented the recommendations from prior pandemic risk assessments (see Chapter 5). For example, the British government stated that the main reason for a nationwide lockdown was to save the National Health Services (NHS) as they are overwhelmed by COVID-19 patients, which explains their motto 'Stay at Home, Protect the NHS, Save Lives'. This lack of NHS capacity was foreseen by many authors who have criticised the government for lack of funding for the NHS, as the annual budget increase did not follow the increase in demand for health-care, and money was spent on expensive services from private health-care companies (El-Gingihy, 2018). Therefore, some have called this pandemic a crisis of governance.

Cognitive dissonance reduction & the sunk cost fallacy: Thus because health services were structurally unprepared to cope with a pandemic, and a severe irreversible pandemic became more and more likely, governments had to suddenly call a state of emergency and had to act with drastic measures such as nationwide lockdowns. To justify their radical measures, they seemed to underline – or even exaggerate – the number of new infections and deaths due to COVID-19, and they kept the worst-case scenario in mind by daily press briefings in the White House or 10 Downing Street. It became politically unfeasible to accept any risks, even when research showed that the pandemic appeared to be severe but not as infectious and fatal as, for example, Ebola. Many opposition parties called to make their political colleagues accountable; for example, in the United Kingdom, a parliamentary committee in the House of Lords started investigating the late and small response to the pandemic by the British government. By isolating individuals, the burden of proof was shifted from the system to particular persons. These governmental responses to the pandemic could be explained as ways to reduce cognitive dissonance. That is, there is a dissonance between the lack of preparation on the one hand and the pandemic and the large-scale governmental responses on the other hand. Politicians will try to close this gap between structural unpreparedness and the current situation. Which strategy they will use will depend on their political situation; for example, opposition members will criticise the government and will call them to resign, whereas members of the government will deny accountability and may point the finger towards others such as foreign governments. However, the underlying problem seemed to be the lack of government preparedness and resilience.

THE CORRUPTION HYPOTHESIS

The history of pandemics is speckled with charlatans. For example, during the 1918 flu pandemic, London newspapers published an advertisement for 'Carbolic Smoke Balls' as a remedy. This was a rubber ball with a tube attached, filled with carbolic acid. The user would insert the tube into their nose and squeeze at the bottom to release the vapours. The nose would run, ostensibly flushing out viral infections. The company behind the carbolic smoke balls was so convinced of their product that they offered £100 to any buyers who became sick. Most likely, they had not imagined any customers would sue them for their claim, but ultimately they lost in court.

Is the COVID-19 pandemic different, and do people not try to take advantage of it? There seem to be some examples of companies and authorities using the situation in their benefit, as we will see in the next chapter. However, although there are some individual cases of cronyism and corruption (Carr, 2020), there seems to be insufficient evidence at this stage to conclude that the pandemic has been completely manipulated or created on a large-scale for the benefit of specific individuals. But it is sure that wealthy investors have been helped and tipped off early in the pandemic by the Trump and Johnson administrations, thanks to which for example party donors have prevented billions in financial losses and have been able to profit from the pandemic by short-selling (wsws.org, 15/10/2020; Huffington Post, 11/10/2020).

The most frequently heard accusation on social media is that the pharmaceutical industry has either caused the pandemic, or that they have influenced the creation of the mechanisms that get triggered when the WHO announces a pandemic. That is, when the WHO communicated on 11 March 2020 that there is a global pandemic, a buying mechanism was automatically triggered which made countries automatically buy vaccinations in advance. For example, the United Kingdom bought vaccines from Glaxo-SmithKline, and the United States from Novarty (Lakoff, 2017). Previously, the WHO has confirmed that their decisions to declare a pandemic were influenced by pharmaceutical companies (ibid.). These observations seem to warrant an investigation. However, it may be premature to argue, like some conspiracy theorists, that because these companies have benefitted from the pandemic they must have caused it. This argument has the same logical structure as the statement that Volkswagen increased its production and innovations due to their involvement with the German national-socialistic regime, and therefore they must have caused the Second World War (correlation/causation conflation fallacy). The reality seems to be that we live in a global empire (Hardt & Negri, 2000). Many companies and institutes try to benefit from any collective crises and pandemics – and even more may lose – but there may not need to be a mega conspiracy behind these mechanisms. If there is governmental misuse, this is more likely to be lower on a sliding scale of corruption (Earle, 2020). Researchers have argued that, if this had been a real conspiracy, there would be so many individuals involved that at least some would have blown the whistle or leaked some information (Keeley, in Uscinski, 2020; Uscinski et al., 2020). Regardless of the extent of the corruption, the fact that some lobbying and influencing had been happening seems to cast some uncertainties over the science and politics of the COVID-19 pandemic.

THE ECOLOGICAL HYPOTHESIS

The world history of pandemics has often been described with three ages of transition (Hardt, 2015). Abdel Omran (1971) writes that pestilence and famine ravaged the Neolithic age, leading to high mortality and low life expectancy, with many infectious diseases, malnutrition, and famine. This era was followed by the age of receding pandemics thanks to modern medicine and more hygienic ways of living, which led to a significant decline in mortality rates and fast population growth. Our current age has seen a fading away of pandemics and an increase in life expectancy. However, it also has seen an increase in new diseases such as cardiovascular diseases, cancer, violence, accidents, and substance abuse – most of which have been attributed to our modern lifestyles and socio-economic inequality (Case & Deaton, 2020; Deaton, 2013).

Although Omran felt certain about his model, he was wrong in predicting that our era would see fewer pandemics. His models had excluded the possibility of change and uncertainties: 'Despite continuing progress in many areas, including enhanced human and animal surveillance and large-scale viral genomic screening, we are probably no better able today to anticipate and prevent the emergence of pandemic influenza than five centuries ago' (Morens et al., 2010). We have entered a new age of pandemics (Quick & Fryer, 2018), with microbes adjusting to our lifestyle and our lifestyle opening new opportunities for their fast transmission (Hardt, 2015). These pandemics are not due to a lack of medicinal expertise, as in the first age, but to an 'outbreak culture' associated with our socio-economic lifestyle (Sabeti & Salahi, 2018). This situation – and the citizens' risk-perceptions – seem to be dominantly shaped by modern politics, and therefore I have elsewhere proposed a fourth age in the world history of health and illness: an era of pandemics caused by our modern economic-political values and lifestyles (Vos, 2020).

These models are examined in our daily life by so-called 'virus-hunters'. Hollywood has cast virology and epidemiology as adventurers in isolated areas and rainforests far away from civilisation. The reality is that tracking down the cause of pandemics is a long-term multidisciplinary effort, which often depends on life-long professional expertise (Keck, 2020; Wolfe, 2011). On the one hand, given the virologic, social, and biological complexity of any pandemic, it is remarkable that researchers have been able to trace the virus to the Wuhan wet market – where rare, live animal species were sold – and to the origins in bats. On the other hand, these hypotheses are not a total surprise, as previous coronaviruses – the relatives of COVID-19 – have been linked to similar markets and species, and thus experts have been using their understanding of this family of viruses to find the ancestor of SARS-CoV-2 (ibid.).

The identification of the environmental cause of COVID-19 needs to be interpreted in the light of the ecological causes of modern pandemics (Vos, 2020; Quammen, 2020). In a recent letter to the US Congress, over 100 wildlife and environmental groups have written that the number of zoonotic diseases has quadrupled over the past 50 years (CoronaVirusWildlifeLetter, 2020). A systematic review indicates that more than half of these are zoonotic diseases associated with agriculture and land-change (Schwab & Malleret, 2020). Thus, it seems that humanity is exposed to more previously unknown viruses due to changes in land use. Most pandemics start with the infection of some wildlife or domestic animal species, which transmit their virus to humans due to living near them or being hunted by them. Although the pathogen cross-over between species seems unpredictable, the likelihood of such crossovers increases because of our lifestyles. For instance, deforestation has increased human contact with unknown animal species, and SARS-Cov and SARS-CoV-2 seem to have come from bats and civets. When we disrupt ecosystems, kill the natural habitat and cage animals for sale, we bring unknown viruses to human society. Climate change has also caused global coverage by Aedes species, such as Zika and dengue mosquitoes, creating pandemics in countries as far north as the United States. The industrial-scale of animal farming has transformed farms into mass factories close to human civilisation, where infections such as foot-and-mouth disease can quickly spread and cross over to humans. The increased demand for livestock and the decreased margins of profit seem to have moti-vated many animal farmers to give antibiotics to their animals, which may have lowered the effectiveness of antibiotics and which may have impacted the human immune system. Areas with severe air pollution may also see more and more severe cases of COVID-19 (Schwab & Malleret, 2020). Scientists also have found that SARS-CoV-2 was spread via wet markets of live animals in Wuhan. Until the 1990s, these markets were small, but wealth expansion has increased the demand for rare animals for culinary dishes that were in the past only imag-inable for the ultra-rich. In sum, our modern (globalist? wealthy? capitalist?) lifestyles seem to have caused the COVID-19 pandemic.

THE HYPER-CONNECTION HYPOTHESIS

We live in a hyper-connected world, with fast developments and complex mechanisms (Schwab & Malleret, 2020). Any simplifying model would be insufficient to explain all causes and responses to the COVID-19 pandemic. Scientists have argued that the virus has been able to spread too fast because the holiday season had just started when the virus affected the first individu-als. Subsequently, the pandemic quickly affected Iran and Italy due to heavy traffic with China, thanks to the One Belt One Road initiative which was an agreement on mutual trade and investment by China in these countries

(Betrus, 2020). In the United States, New York was specifically affected, as was London in the United Kingdom; scientists have explained the large infection rates in these cities by the fact that these are very multicultural cities with international flight hubs (ibid.). Thus, it seems that the hyper-connectedness of our world has played a significant role in the spread of the virus. In sum, globalisation and multicultural societies may not come without risks.

THE CAPITALISM HYPOTHESIS

The previous sections discussed the role of modern governmental risk management, corruption, ecological crisis, and hyper-connection. If one imagines these as dots in a connect-the-dots image, which image would emerge? When I connected these dots in a previous book, the image of capitalism – more specifically neoliberalism – emerged. For example, over 6,000 articles were published in scientific journals on COVID-19, which I will discuss in the following sections. My previous book on *The Economics of Meaning in Life* analysed how the economic system determines what individual citizens experience as meaningful in life (Vos, 2020). In line with other authors, I argue that the governmental approach to the pandemic further stimulated the capitalist lifestyle and the capitalist way of thinking (Mezzadri, 2020; Žižek, 2020). In my book I argue that neoliberalism brings a unique combination of perspectives on life, including materialism, self-orientedness and functionalism. This combination seems to underlie some of the government decisions during the COVID-19 pandemic, and this pandemic also seems to enforce and reinforce a materialist, self-oriented and functionalist perspective on citizens. Furthermore, I found overall empirical evidence for the hypothesis that capitalism and COVID-19 are related. A systematic review found a moderately strong correlation between the capitalistic characteristics of a country and the number of infections and deaths related to COVID-19 (Vos, 2020). It seems that the more capitalist a country is, the more people may get infected and die; this does not seem surprising, given this combination of biopolitics, prioritising numbers of people and growing inequality, as the next sections will show.

THE BIOPOLITICS HYPOTHESIS

The *European Journal of Psychoanalysis* published a debate between modern philosophers about the biopolitics of COVID-19. The editors argued that to understand the psychological interpretation and impact of COVID-19, we need to understand how politics and biology have got more and more interwoven during the last centuries.

Biopower: The journal started with a publication by the philosopher Michel Foucault from the 1970s, who popularised the term 'biopolitics'. With this term, he referred to a 'set of mechanisms through which the basic biological features of the human species became the object of a political strategy, of a general strategy of power, or, in other words, how, starting from the 18th century, modern Western societies took on board the fundamental biological fact that human beings are a species'. This involves an intricate apparatus of subjugating bodies and exerting control over an entire population or global mass. Governments regulate all aspects of life, from birth to death, production, and illness; as such, they create a generalised functionalistic society. The aim is not merely to make individuals behave, to be efficient and productive workers, but to manage a total population and ensure a healthy workforce. Thus, governments have moved towards mass management of human bodies via behaviour control technologies from disciplines such as economics, biology, virology, epidemiology, sociology, and psychology. The focus is no longer on how to govern people – as sovereigns like kings and nobility did in the past – but to organise life on a larger scale and make people conform to the prescribed safety behaviour. Like Deleuze (1995) wrote: we have moved from societies of discipline – where discipline was taught in schools, factories, or hospitals – to societies of control with mobile, flexible networks of existence.

'We saw the emergence of techniques of power that were essentially centred on the body, on the individual body. They included all devices that were used to ensure the spatial distribution of individuals' bodies (their separation, their alignment, their serialization, and their surveillance) and the organization, around those individuals, of a whole field of visibility. They were also techniques that could be used to take control over bodies. Attempts were made to increase their productive force through exercise, drill, and so on. They were also techniques for rationalizing and strictly economizing on a power that had to be used in the least costly way possible, thanks to whole systems of surveillance, hierarchies, inspections, book-keeping, and reports – all the technology of labour. It was established at the end of the seventeenth century, and in the course of the eighteenth century.'

Surveillance: Many authors have criticised governments for their biopolitical use of surveillance technologies to control the population during COVID-19. This includes the test-and-trace system that many countries have put in place, which has raised questions over data security (Cosgrove et al., 2020; French & Monahan, 2020; Kitchin, 2020; Mühlhoff, 2020; Westoby & Harris, 2020).

Other authors have argued that governments may use this situation as a shock doctrine, as politicians may try to enforce policies that citizens would usually protest against but they may feel too shocked to do so now; later sections will elaborate on this (Gürcan & Kahraman, 2020).

Exclusion: Foucault describes how, during medieval pandemics, sick individuals were either disciplined – locked at home or in hospitals – or excluded from society, for instance being sent to leper colonies. After the pandemic, patients may have died or survived, but the governmental technologies seemed to remain in place. Imposing control and exclusion became a habit for politicians in other groups as well: the role of the leper was substituted by the poor, by vagrants, by prisoners, and by those considered 'mad' who were now excluded. This mechanism of exclusion that started with pandemics has become a key feature of modern biopolitics. Consequently, when confronted with risks, uncertainties or deviations from the norm, modern politicians seem inclined to think in terms of exclusion, lockup, or lockdown, combined with mass surveillance. As guards were checking at the city gates whether newcomers had symptoms of the plague, during COVID-19 newcomers are checked for fever or for using hand gel and face-masks by border guards, bus drivers, police officers and security officers at the entrance of pubs, restaurants, and stores.

The exclusion/inclusion mechanisms seem to have split society: those who are included – the hierarchy, accepted by the health authorities via surveillance, observation, and test-and-trace – versus those who are excluded, outcasts, the sick, etc. Like governments use generalising names for groups such as 'the keyworkers', 'the sick', 'the elderly' and 'the vulnerable', by reifying these categories, they create exclusive groups. This does not seem to do justice to the complexity of the subjectively lived experiences of individuals. This unrealistic, dehumanised approach of citizens became significant when the British and American governments used the mathematical a-psychological models of Ferguson to impose nationwide lockdowns. Consequently, the mathematical exclusion mechanisms have socially transformed our cities, villages, and neighbourhoods. In the Middle Ages, political exclusion transformed plague towns into 'segmented, immobile, frozen spaces, each fixed in his place', with public squares and markets devoid of social interactions except for the frightening figure of the plague-doctor in his black suit and his black beak filled with anti-viral herbs. This medieval dystopia of the plague town has uncanny resemblances with the empty streets in Wuhan and countless other cities across the globe, with body-suited medicals and citizens hiding their looks out of fear for their potentially infectious or potentially infectable fellow-humans behind their face-masks.

Necropolitics: Biopolitics is Foucault's depiction of the modern assessment and control of life across the population. Biopolitics aims at creating the best conditions for the survival of the many, putting the preservation of mere biological life above economic or political well-being. This means that governments do not focus on the citizen's individual right to life, but on all lives – Life (with a capital) in general.

The Italian philosophers Agamben and Esposito have argued that the abstract concept of biological life has become sacred in modern societies and that this has replaced the inherent meaningfulness of an individual life. Consequently, to save Life in general, the lives of individuals may need to be sacrificed, like Adolf Hitler justified the Final Solution – the extinction of individual Jews – to save humankind. Esposito calls this process 'social immunisation'. That is, when a doctor gives a patient an immunisation shot, the patient gets a small version of the evil that the vaccination should prevent, such as flu. A little bit of illness is needed to save health. Some deaths may also be needed – as in rare circumstances vaccinations could have negative side effects – to save the life of the population in general.

Thus, biopolitics seems to involve necropolitics ('necro' regards death) inherently. Achille Mbembe (2019) writes that necropolitics does not only involve the right to kill, but also the right to expose individuals – including a country's citizens – to suffering, illness, and death. This includes the right for authorities to impose social or civil death, the right of enslavement and other forms of creating 'walking dead'. Legal impunity is given to anyone responsible for causing illnesses, severe side effects, and the deaths of individuals, as long as they may have saved biological life in the population in general. For example, during the COVID-19 pandemic, several Western countries have argued that they did not want to go into lockdown. However, they wanted to create herd immunity, which means the natural process – without vaccinations – whereby some individuals in the population get sick, and by overcoming their disease, they develop antibodies and become naturally immune. If enough people develop herd immunity, the pandemic should halt. However, herd immunity implies that many people will get sick, and some may die; as the British Prime Minister said: 'many families will lose loved ones'. The death of the individual is an acceptable price for the immunity of the herd.

Similarly, the physical and psychological side effects of the lockdowns – including suicides and deaths from postponed non-COVID-19-related medical consultations and surgeries – seem to be widely accepted without much public outcry – as the bigger picture is saving Life in General. Several governments have withheld the publication of the number of deaths of health-care workers – as if their deaths are irrelevant when seen from the bigger picture of stopping the pandemic. Another clear example is the WHO guideline which says that researchers and pharmaceutical companies are not liable for any deaths or other side effects of vaccinations during pandemics – as stopping the pandemic is more important than preventing individual suffering.

Agamben (2020a, 2020b) writes how this governmental necropolitics excludes certain individuals from society, in the name of naked Biological Life. Agamben compares these excluded individuals with the *Homo Sacer* in Roman law. The *Homo Sacer* was an individual who could be killed without punishment, as their death was regarded as beneficial for the society in general. What matters is not saving the life of one individual, but the abstract concept of Life in general. To apply Agamben's ideas: although the British government let go of the option of herd immunity – due to political pressure and quickly rising infection and mortality rates – and they imposed a nationwide lockdown, their focus seemed to remain unchanged. That is, the British motto 'Stay at Home, Protect the NHS, Save Lives' shows that the final goal of the pandemic management is to save the abstract concept of lives – not the specific life of John, my elderly neighbour, but Lives in general. Naturally, this is a simplistic criticism, as governments need to generalise their policies and they cannot name each individual impacted by their policies. However, to achieve their goal of stopping the pandemic, the press conferences made clear that individuals need to sacrifice their individual well-being – their body and psyche – by staying at home. Seen from a larger perspective: instead of offering a well-functioning state apparatus which could save lives – such as well-preparing and well-funding the NHS – the government admits in their slogan that they only have one aim: solving their failure to prepare the NHS: 'Save the NHS'. Subsequently, the government seems to shift the responsibility away from themselves to individual citizens and makes them responsible for saving the NHS and saving lives. In terms of Agamben, the previously created weakness of the NHS seems to have enabled the government to create *Homo Sacers* and to enact their exclusionary policies.

To exemplify the necropolitics during COVID-19: several authors have criticised governments for prioritising numbers over people. They have pointed at the dehumanised ways of communication – for example, in the daily press briefings from the White House or 10 Downing Street, impersonal infection and mortality figures were communicated (De Genova, 2020; Fuchs, 2020; Sobande, 2020). It has been argued that the message 'we are all in this together' was hiding money-focused and commodified concepts of human connection, care and community. Examples include the rejection of governments to prepare for future pandemics despite reports warning about a lack of PPE and ventilators, slow production due to monopolies on the market, researchers not sharing scientific expertise to keep a competitive advantage, and financial dependence of researchers and health organisations on grants/donations from pharmaceutical companies and Big Capital (Vos, 2020). Furthermore, governmental communication has been criticised for hiding research reports on the unequal impact of COVID-19, as individuals with low socio-economic status, Black people and ethnic minorities are more likely to get infected and to develop severe forms of COVID-19 (see below). This has been described as racial capitalism, replicating historical inequities within pandemics, and not improving access for these groups to adequate health resources (Della Rosa & Goldstein, 2020; Pirtle, 2020). Agamben summarises this point as follows:

'The first thing the wave of panic that's paralysed the country has clearly shown is that our society no longer believes in anything but naked life. It is evident that [we] are prepared to sacrifice practically everything – normal living conditions, social relations, work, even friendships and religious or political beliefs – to avoid the danger of falling ill. The naked life, and the fear of losing it, is not something that brings men and women together, but something that blinds and separates them. Other human beings, like those in the plague described by Manzoni, are now seen only as potential contaminators to be avoided at all costs or at least to keep at a distance of at least one metre. The dead – our dead – have no right to a funeral and it's not clear what happens to the corpses of our loved ones. Our fellow humans have been erased and it's odd that the Churches remain silent on this point. What will human relations become in a country that will be accustomed to living in this way for who knows how long? And what is a society with no other value other than survival?'

The chapter on mental health will give some examples of how human beings are reduced to naked life, as stigma seems to be one of the largest concerns of patients and frontline workers. For example, health-care workers describe that they feel excluded by their friends and relatives, as they are afraid that they may be infected; others treat them as if they are stripped from all their subjective experiences, anxieties, and grief. There are occasional reports of physical assaults on health-care workers and police officers during the pandemic. Meanwhile, the health-care worker has been described as 'Superman' by the ministers and secretaries of the British government; this symbol of Superman seems to strip them from their subjectivity, their personal experiences and needs as if they are a League of Avengers that is beyond any human needs such as sufficient PPE and a pay rise. They have become naked life ('zoe'), and not individuals in the political community (bios) with their own unique voice and meaningfulness (logos) (Agamben, 2020a, 2020b).

Governmentality during COVID-19 (technologies of the market): Foucault writes that there are in general two types of biopolitics: those that focus on directly governing the people, for example by imposing rules and laws, and those that focus on stimulating citizens to govern themselves such as making them feel responsible, guilty and ashamed about their health behaviour. The clearest example of governmentality is imposing a lockdown and having police and soldiers patrol the streets, and fine or imprison offenders. The emergency acts that parliaments in several countries have approved have given much power to the government, police, and army in controlling the people. These acts have been criticised by human rights organisations who argue that the powers are too broad, that there is not sufficient democratic control and accountability, and that the time limit is too long – for example, two years in the UK (Human Rights Watch, 2020). Not only may these governmentality strategies impinge on democratic principles, they may also be difficult and expensive to enforce. For example, there may not be enough police officers and soldiers to control whether each citizen is staying at home and always using PPE.

Several sociologists have argued that the relative increase in powers of the executive – the government – has been a gradual but strong trend in countries across the globe during the last decades (Rosanvallon, 2018). This comes at the cost of decreased powers for parliaments and the judiciary. For example, COVID-19 emergency bills give governments more powers to act without consultation by parliament. The new legislation was also announced quickly, without sufficient time for courts to develop jurisprudence and to test the emergency laws on the constitution – which had created embarrassing moments for governments when judges overruled certain parts of the emergency bills in individual court rulings. Thus, COVID-19 seems to be the result and the acceleration of a fundamental crisis in democracy. This disbalance between the executive, legislative and judiciary powers seems to be related to the increased powers of the traditional and social media as well as the increased use of self-govermentality strategies, as will be explained below (Vos, 2020).

Self-governmentality during COVID-19 (technologies of the self): In recent centuries, increased medical expertise, wealth, and hygiene have improved life expectancies across the globe. This implied that large-scale governmental interventions were no longer needed and that the focus of action moved to the individual citizen, albeit nudged by their governments. This meant that more subtle and rational mechanisms were introduced, such as a self-help culture, private insurances, individual and collective savings, safety measures such as

PPE for sale to individuals on Amazon and Ebay, and so on. Individual citizens gradually acquiesce to subtle regulations and expectations of the social order: they internalise norms and values and take responsibility for managing their risks via safety behaviours – such as buying their own masks and deciding to self-isolate or to go out.

Foucault argues that this internalisation of governmental norms and values mainly happens via 'regimes of truth', such as the traditional and social media that shape our perception and behaviour – elaborated in the next chapters. For example, the daily briefings in the White House and 10 Downing Street did not merely relay medical facts; they also seemed to tell citizens what to think, how to feel and what to do. Individuals would no longer stay at home merely because they were told to do so, but they felt guilty or ashamed if they did not do so. This led to paradoxical messages from governments such as: 'you are allowed to go outside, but you still need to be careful out there.' These paradoxical messages would trigger so many health worries in people, that they would govern themselves by staying inside, even despite the legal ability to go to pubs or restaurants. This self-governmentality became particularly visible with the online shaming of 'covidiots' (see Chapter 5).

Self-governmentality can involve multiple processes. *Responsibilisation* means that citizens start to feel responsible for tasks which were previously considered the responsibility of the state. *Normalisation* entails, for example, the acceptance of what has been called 'the new normal'. For example, hearing daily figures about COVID-19 infections and deaths also seemed to numb people, and numbers seemed to feel normal. *Healthism* links the 'public objectives for the good health and good order of the social body with the desire of individuals for health and well-being' (Rose, 1999, p.74). The latter means that the state does not seek to discipline, instruct, moralise, or threaten citizens into compliance, but it addresses citizens on the assumption that they are motivated themselves to be healthy and to take care of their health. This has stimulated the rise of countless health experts – including self-acclaimed experts lacking external recognition of their expertise – as reflected in the flurry of social media posts.

Finally, self-governmentality also seems to include *self-exclusion and self-sacrifice* for the sake of naked Biological Life. For many individuals, self-isolation has had high financial, physical, psychological and social costs, but when asked in polls, they answer that they would do it again, even when self-isolation was not needed to save the population (see Chapter 8). It seems that all side effects – including suicide – have become justified if the abstract concept of Life in general can be saved. Citizens have been transformed from individuals with a voice in the democratic processes of the political community (*zoe*) and their subjective meanings (*logos*) to naked biological life (*zoe*). They are no longer individual citizens, but potential bombs loaded with the COVID-19 virus against which the population should be protected. Furthermore, self-governmentality has turned these potential bombs inwards, as individuals have become obsessed with themselves and their own feelings of guilt, shame and anxiety.

Totalitarianism: Several authors have compared some of the responses to the COVID-19 pandemic with totalitarianism. One of the strongest formulations on 'Covidian Cult' has possibly been voiced by Hopkins (*Consentfactory. org*, 13/10/2020):

'One of the hallmarks of totalitarianism is mass conformity to a psychotic official narrative. Not a regular official narrative, like the "Cold War" or the "War on Terror" narratives. A totally delusional official narrative that has little or no connection to reality and that is contradicted by a preponderance of facts. Nazism and Stalinism are the classic examples, but the phenomenon is better observed in cults and other sub-cultural societal groups. (…) Looking in from the dominant culture (or back through time in the case of the Nazis), the delusional nature of these official narratives is glaringly obvious to most rational people. What many people fail to understand is that to those who fall prey to them (whether individual cult members or entire totalitarian societies) such narratives do not register as psychotic. On the contrary, they feel entirely normal. Everything in their social "reality" reifies and reaffirms the narrative, and anything that challenges or contradicts it is perceived as an existential threat. These narratives are invariably paranoid, portraying the cult as threatened or persecuted by an evil enemy or antagonistic force which only unquestioning conformity to the cult's ideology can save its members from. (…) In addition to being paranoid, these narratives are often internally inconsistent, illogical, and … well, just completely ridiculous. This does not weaken them, as one might suspect. Actually, it increases their power, as it forces their adherents to attempt to reconcile their inconsistency and irrationality, and in many cases utter absurdity, in order to remain in good standing with the cult. Such reconciliation is of course impossible, and causes the cult members' minds to short circuit and abandon any semblance of critical thinking, which is precisely what the cult leader wants. (…)

It is happening to most of our societies right now. An official narrative is being implemented. A totalitarian official narrative. A totally psychotic official narrative, no less delusional than that of the Nazis, or the Manson family, or any other cult. Most people cannot see that it is happening, for the simple reason that it is happening to them. They are literally unable to recognize it.

The human mind is extremely resilient and inventive when it is pushed past its limits. When reality falls apart completely, the mind will create a delusional narrative, which appears just as "real" as our normal reality, because even a delusion is better than the stark raving terror of utter chaos. And this is why so many people – people who are able to easily recognize totalitarianism in cults and foreign countries – cannot perceive the totalitarianism that is taking shape now, right in front of their faces (or, rather, right inside their minds). Nor can they perceive the delusional nature of the official "Covid-19" narrative, no more than those in Nazi Germany were able to perceive how completely delusional their official "master race" narrative was. Such people are neither ignorant nor stupid. They have been successfully initiated into a cult, which is essentially what totalitarianism is, albeit on a societal scale. Their initiation into the Covidian Cult began in January, when the medical authorities and corporate media turned on The Fear. The global masses have been subjected to a constant stream of propaganda, manufactured hysteria, wild specula-tion, conflicting directives, exaggerations, lies, and tawdry theatrical effects. Lockdowns. Emergency field hospitals and morgues. The singing-dancing NHS staff. Death trucks. Overflowing ICUs. Dead Covid babies. Manipulated statistics. Goon squads. Masks. And all the rest of it.

While it is crucial to continue reporting the facts and sharing them with as many people as possible – which is becoming increasingly difficult due to the censorship of alternative and social media – it is important to accept what we are up against. What we are up against is not a misunderstanding or a rational argument over scientific facts. It is a fanatical ideological movement. A global totalitarian movement … the first of its kind in human history. Instead of the cult existing as an island within the dominant culture, the cult has become the dominant culture, and those of us who have not joined the cult have become the isolated islands within it.'

THE STATE OF EXCEPTION AND THE SHOCK DOCTRINE HYPOTHESIS

> 'Governemnts love pandemics. They love pandemics for the same reason they love war. Because it gives them the ability to impose controls on the popula-tion that the population would otherwise never accept. To create institutions and mechanisms for orchestrating and imposing obedience.' (Robert Kennedy, Berlin, 29/08/2020).

Whereas Foucault saw the mechanisms of control and exclusion as a rare modern phenomenon, Giorgio Agamben (2017) writes about the tendency for governments to use a state of exception as a normal paradigm. For example, whereas governments introduced large-scale surveillance as exceptional after 9/11 this may have now become normal. While the public rescue of banks after the 2007/8 crash was coined as exceptional, this has happened many times again. Agamben (2020a, 2020b) sees the state of exception – 'the new normal'– that was introduced with COVID-19 as part of a larger trend:

> *'The epidemic is clearly showing that the state of exception, which governments began to accustom us to years ago, has become an authentically normal condition. There have been more serious epidemics in the past, but no one ever thought of declaring a state of emergency like today, one that forbids us even to move. Men have become so used to living in conditions of permanent crisis and emergency that they don't seem to notice that their lives have been reduced to a purely biological condition, one that has lost not only any social and political dimension, but even any compassionate and emotional one. A society that lives in a permanent state of emergency cannot be a free one. We effectively live in a society that has sacrificed freedom to so-called "security reasons" and as a consequence has condemned itself to living in a permanent state of fear and insecurity.'*

Not only is the governmental response during COVID-19 a result of the normal political process of states of exception, Agamben also argues that the 'invention of an epidemic offered the ideal pretext' for further limitations to fundamental freedoms. Where 9/11 did not give complete permanent control over citizens, COVID-19 may give the ideal pretext to achieve this.

Naomi Klein (2007) provides a relatively similar argument in her 'disaster capitalism hypothesis'. She describes disaster capitalism as 'the way private industries spring up directly profits from large-scale crisis'. Instead of being a side effect of capitalism, she sees this as a fundamental characteristic of capitalism, in line with Milton Friedman's saying 'only a crisis – actual or perceived – produces real change. When that crisis occurs, government actions depend on the ideas that are lying around. That, I believe, is our basic function: to develop alternatives to existing policies, to keep them alive and available until the politically impossible becomes politically inevitable.' Klein has described the COVID-19 pandemic as such a 'shock doctrine' from which disaster capitalism will benefit – without saying that capitalists have deliberately caused the pandemic.

> *'The crises are actual. We are seeing a very selective use of emergency measures, of the utilization and the instrumentalization and the weaponization of states of emergency to offload risks onto individual workers and families, while the people who are already most cushioned are getting these no-strings-attached bailouts.*

(…) Our daily caloric intake is being delivered to us by Amazon or DoorDash. All of these gig employees who are doing the work are incredibly vulnerable. We are getting a glimpse of the world that Silicon Valley would like to deliver to us and it isn't the way we want to live. We don't want our social lives to be mineable, survey-able. This is the future that Silicon Valley has in store for us. I think we should in a sense see this as an opportunity to refuse that future in the way that we come out of this crisis.(…) We can see the grotesque economic divisions widening further. We are trying to deal with the impacts of the pandemic within the fallout, within the rubble of the austerity policies of the foreclosure crisis, and the decimation of labour standards that grew out of the last crisis.(…) Normal is deadly. We don't need to stimulate the economy. We need to build an economy that is based on protecting lives.' (InTheseTimes, 27/03/2020)

Can COVID-19 indeed be regarded as an example of disaster capitalism? Several thinkers have argued that the supposed 'state of exception' or 'shock doctrine' has not been applied everywhere. For example, China and Italy imposed a lockdown, but the UK and US delayed this for a long time and Sweden did not have a lockdown. Furthermore, even the most neoliberal governments have agreed on large stimulus packages to support the most vulnerable in societies and to stimulate the economy. We should also be careful with building explanations like these, as there may be a risk of confirmation bias when a theory of long-running processes is used as a framework for a recent not-totally-unfolded event. We could, for example, instead see governments as nothing more than grim executioners and taking it out on them may be more like a diversionary manoeuvre than sincere political reflection (Nancy, 2020).

Regardless of the extent to which capitalists may use the pandemic for profit, some politicians and private companies may make use of the uncertainties of the pandemic. For example, the president of the World Economic Forum, Schwab, has argued that COVID-19 will offer the 'Great Reset' that society needs in his opinion. This has led to some criticasters to accuse him of 'fascism', as he wants to use the pandemic to enforce his own political-economic agenda – a larger role for private businesses and an increased technologization of society, bypassing parliament (e.g. WinterOak, 5/10/2020). He had already announced before the start of the pandemic that the theme of the next forum in Davos would be the 'Great Reset' and that they would need to reflect on how they could achieve this restart of the economic system:

'[The pandemic] could go beyond a mere acceleration by altering things that previously seemed unchangeable. It might thus provoke changes that would have seemed inconceivable before the pandemic struck, such as new forms of monetary policy like helicopter money (already given), the reconsideration/recalibration

of some of our social priorities and an augmented search for the common good as a policy objective, the notion of fairness acquiring political potency, radical welfare and taxation measures, and drastic geopolitical realignments. The possibilities for change and the resulting new order are now unlimited and only bound by our imagination, for better or for worse. Societies could be poised to become either more egalitarian or more authoritarian or geared towards more solidarity or individualism, favouring the interests of the few or the many. We should take advantage of this unprecedented opportunity to reimagine our world, in a bid to make it a better and more resilient one as it emerges on the other side of this crisis.' (Schwab & Malleret, 2020, p.18)

INEQUALITY MODELS

Perhaps we should not speak about pandemics, but about supersyndemics. Supersyndemics describe the synergy – that is, accumulation, interaction or mediation – of two or more conditions. A supersyndemic is the combination of a medical pandemic like COVID-19 with other factors. 'In short, health and wealth go hand in hand, and as a result, the poor have worse health than the more affluent social groups. The chief underlying cause of health disparities is increasingly understood to be social and economic inequality, i.e., social conditions that either directly produce ill health or promote unhealthy behaviours that lead to poor health' (Singer, 2009, p.xiii). Thus, the political mantra 'we are all in this together' seems to brush away painful healthy diversities. Consequently, it is unlikely that solutions for the pandemics are one-size-fits-all, as it needs to address a wide variety of variations and factors. We should look at epidemiology with a social gaze and not merely with a biomedical gaze (Berkman et al., 2014; O'Campo & Dunn, 2011).

Socio-economic class: In the previous decade, 'there has been an explosion of research indicating that social class is a powerful, and arguably the most powerful, predictor of health' (Budrys, 2003, p.181). Many pandemics in the past, such as tuberculosis, seem to be concentrated among the poor. In recent years, we have also seen a staggering increase of so-called 'deaths of despair' from suicide, drug overdose, and alcoholism, which are associated with people's low socio-economic status and low social mobility (Case & Deaton, 2020; Deaton, 2013).

COVID-19 does not seem to be an exception to these research findings. People come from uneven starting points into this pandemic, with individuals in the most socio-economically deprived areas more likely to have chronic conditions that put them at a greater risk of developing a severe form of COVID-19. Consequently, COVID-19 seems to infect individuals with a lower socio-economic status more frequently and with more severe symptoms than those with a higher status (*Intensive Care National Audit Research Centre*, 20/07/2020; BBC News, 12/04/2020). However, governments have been refusing to publish reports on the health inequalities of COVID-19 (*IFS Deaton Review*, 18/10/2020).

During the nationwide lockdown, individuals with low socio-economic status were more likely to be exposed to high-risk situations as their work is outdoors, examples being manual workers, waste collectors, supermarket staff, postal delivery services, police officers, nurses, cleaning personnel, etc. The poorest are the most likely to work during quarantine (Bibby et al., 2020). This increases their risk of infection, and governments are still refusing to publish data on how many frontline workers have died from COVID-19 (*Guardian*, 16/04/2020). Furthermore, quarantine may be less effective, or even detrimental, when people live in small overcrowded housing conditions, which increases the risk of the virus spreading. Other socio-economic factors also make individuals from a low socio-economic background more at risk, such as having less money to buy vitamin-rich food and greater psychological stress which could create an impaired immune system that could result in more severe cases of COVID-19 (Berkman et al., 2014; O'Campo & Dunn, 2011; Singer, 2009; Marmot, 2001; Marmot & Wilkinson, 2005).

Economic impact: Before the COVID-19 pandemic, the world economy has never come to such an abrupt stop and drastic and dramatic collapse (Schwab & Malleret, 2020). This economic impact has mainly been the result of governments deciding to go into nationwide or regional lockdowns, which hypothetically could slow down or even halt the transmission. According to the OECD, the largest economies will most likely see a reduction in GDP between 20% and 30% (oecd.org, 10/06/2020). According to one economic model, an economic hibernation of the Dutch economy for one month would mean a shrinkage of 1.2% (cpb.nl, March 2020). From all economies, the United States has been hit the hardest: for example, in March and April, 36 million Americans lost their jobs, reversing ten years of job gains, as companies could easily make them redundant in their hire-and-fire culture. The pandemic may also lead to structural economic changes, such as staff – mainly manual labourers – being replaced with robots and intelligent machines which cannot get sick (Schwab & Malleret, 2020).

The long-term economic impact that COVID-19 may have will depend on the duration and severity of the outbreak, the success of containing the pandemic and mitigating its effects, and the cohesiveness of society when the physical isolation is over (ibid.). However, these factors are still uncertain, and consequently, the long-term impact on the economies of the world, nations and our household remain uncertain for now. The IMF summarised the situation in its World Economic Outlook in June 2020 with two words: 'uncertain recovery'. Much is still uncertain, even whether there will be deflation or inflation. What is certain is that the ripple effects on employment and economic growth may last several years – or even decades – and may interact with other uncertain factors such as declining populations and Brexit (ibid.).

However, 'the socio-economic impact of the pandemic does not seem to be borne equally by different echelons of society. Although many parliaments have quickly passed emergency bills to allocate large sums of money to support those hit hardest by COVID-19, they have been criticised for offering too little too late – only temporarily covering some of the first economic impacts. Some of these bills, such as the emergency Covid-19 Legislation in the United Kingdom, include clauses that strengthen the powers of employers, for example, to lay off staff, which politicians argue is crucial for the economy' (Vos, 2020, p.312). While at the one end of the socio-economic spectrum, one-quarter of the full Western population may file for unemployment – the biggest unemployment ever measured (Armstrong, 2020; VOXEU, 16/05/2020; Metro, 12/10/2020), at the other end are those individuals who have benefited from the pandemic. As one investor said: 'When there are fear and increased uncertainty in the market, which is what shorter-term investors focus on, we find there is a great opportunity' (ProActive Investors UK, 05/03/2020). COVID-19 has offered profitable business opportunities to COVID-19-related companies such as pharmacy chains, Novacyt PLC – the monopolist on the Primedesign diagnostic tests – and companies like Reckitt producing disinfectants and PPE. The lockdown also boosted takeaway food companies, postal delivery services such as Amazon, services such as Zoom and Microsoft, and home entertainment such as Netflix and Disney Plus (Betrus, 2020; Vos, 2020). Thus, the COVID-19 pandemic may not be the big equaliser that some people claim it is, but it seems to be the big un-equaliser of our era.

Race: 'There is nothing new for us', Theopia Jackson said at the IMEC International Meaning Conference 2019. Jackson is an expert on health diversity, and she was asked to speak about the Black Lives Matter movement in relation to COVID-19. She explained how the unequal impact of the pandemic on Black people is in line with countless studies, which she explained as follows: 'When a white person coughs once, we are sick.' In general, infectious diseases seem to infect disproportionally large numbers of Black people and with greater severity. We see the same during the COVID-19 pandemic. Almost all of the US kids and teens who have died from COVID-19 were Hispanic or Black (CDC, 14/09/2020). For example, in Chicago, more than 50% of

COVID-19 cases and nearly 70% of COVID-19 deaths involve Black individuals, although they make up only 30% of the population (Yancy, 2020). 'The excess deaths among African-Americans "are shining a very bright light on some of the real weaknesses and foibles in our society," said Anthony Fauci, director of the National Institute of Allergy and Infectious Diseases, adding that at least part of the problem was due to a higher burden of underlying medical conditions such as diabetes, hypertension, obesity, and asthma among African-Americans. "There's nothing we can do about it right now except to try and give them the best possible care to avoid complications," he said' (Dyer, 2020, p.1). These findings of an unequal impact on Black individuals have been replicated across the globe (e.g. Price-Haywood et al., 2020; Laurencin & McClinton, 2020).

Global inequality: We have not been able to fathom the long-term economic impact of COVID-19 on the world's most vulnerable communities. Countries with limited infrastructure and basic health-care already seem to be struggling in containing the pandemic (see the discussion in the next chapter on vertical and horizontal aid). The reduced demand for products in the West may lead to unemployment down the supply chain to the producers, small farmers, and factory workers (Schwab & Malleret, 2020). We may also start to see a trend of regionalisation of economies in response to the assumed health dangers of global transport and flights. Thus, it seems time to rethink pandemics as pathologies of socio-economic and political power (Farmer, 2003). We need to look 'upstream' to identify and tackle the social determinants of health (Ratcliff, 2017).

> *'In life-and-death matters such as the COVID-19 pandemic, a focus on financial matters can seem misplaced. But for the world's poor, the financial impacts of COVID-19 can be devastating and far more immediate.'* (Tarazi, CGAP.com)

HOW TO CREATE RESILIENT POLITICS

All pandemics are political, according to Carol who I interviewed for this book. This seems to be a good summary of this chapter which started with describing how governments may have acted to prevent serious irreversible damage, trying to avoid any risks and particularly the worst-case scenario, shifting the burden of proof to others while they were unprepared and stuck to previous policies to save their faces and voters. There is clear evidence that the pandemic was influenced or exacerbated by a global ecological collapse, global hyper-connection, capitalism, and some influences from the pharmaceutical industry and other commercial actors. Thus, this pandemic seems to be highly political: the difference between biology and politics seems to have become blurred. It is in this political and socio-economic context that individual citizens develop their own perceptions of the pandemic, and decide which precautions to take – if any at all.

Many authors seem to paint the pandemic with a Janus face and it is uncertain which will dominate. On the one face, there are those arguing how biopolitics undermines the material, psychological and social conditions of individual empowerment, democracy and revolution. On the other face, there are those saying that the pandemic is motivating people to reflect, criticise and rise against authoritarian governments. These changing attitudes seem to stand in a longer trend: since the 2007/8 financial crisis, the public support for capitalism is rapidly decreasing (Vos, 2020; Ostry et al., 2016; Bowman & Rugg, 2013; Atkinson & Elliott, 2008). People are shifting away from the materialist, self-oriented and functionalistic approaches towards social and larger types of meaning in life (Vos, 2020). A similar trend is visible for COVID-19: several authors have described that COVID-19 has put capitalism on a crossroads, as the pandemic – and particularly the lockdown – has made citizens reflect on their values in life and economic priorities (Murshed, 2020; Saad-Filho, 2020; Schwab & Malleret, 2020). Several authors show how the pandemic has triggered calls from politicians and political activists to use this crisis to overturn the capitalist mindset, with proposals such as universal basic income, egalitarian distribution of goods, free health-care and public funding for research (Nelson, 2020; San Juan, 2020; Shamasunder et al., 2020). They show how a human rights movement is growing (Smith, 2020), as the journalist Gabriel Tupinamba wrote (in Žižek, 2020, p.135):

'I really can feel something heroic about this new ethics – everybody works day and night from their home office, participating in video conferences and taking care of children or schooling them at the same time, but nobody asks why he or she is doing it, because it's not any more a question of so 'I get money and can go to vacation etc.', since nobody knows if there will be vacations again and if there will be money. It's the idea of a world where you have an apartment, basics like food and water, the love of others and a task that really matters, now more than ever. The idea that one needs "more" seems unreal now.'

To build resilient politics to prepare for future pandemics involves both individual and collective activities. Individuals could develop their critical thinking skills, for example via higher education. They could also educate themselves on how the political system influences them, and where logical critical questions could be asked – without falling into the trap of conspiracy theories. On a collective scale, imbalances in the political system due to exorbitant executive powers should be prevented via the constitution and the independence of the judiciary. States of exception should possibly only be allowed under democratic scrutiny, clear accountability procedures and with strict time limits. Individual citizens should be protected from political and commercial powers using pandemics as a shock-doctrine to push through any controversial policies, for example by increased transparency of decision-making and strict anti-corruption rules. New laws could clearly define the political exclusions that politicians can make, and which they cannot make, during states of exception, such as reflecting on the costs of human lives when governments do not lockdown but go for herd immunity, and alternatively on the costs of lockdown. Scientists should have a more critical role during pandemics, independent from politicians and pharmaceutical companies and other commercial actors. Finally, COVID-19 could be a wake-up call to address these issues around ecological collapse, increased vulnerability due to hyper-connectedness and biopower.

4

MEDIA RISKS

UNCERTAIN JOURNALISTS

'In an ever-changing, incomprehensible world, the masses had reached the point where they would at the same time, believe everything and nothing, think that everything was possible and nothing was true.' (Arendt, 1973, p.87)

OVERVIEW

What do the following statements have in common? Coronavirus Vaccines Contain Nanotechnology Microchips to Control Humans. Vodka Can Be Used As Hand Sanitiser. Eating Garlic Prevents Coronavirus. Netflix launched COVID-19 to promote its new series. Drinking Cow Urine Protects Against Covid-19. Russia Have Released Lions To Enforce Social Distancing. Answer: all these statements are not fringe-ideas advocated only by small groups, but newspapers have printed these ideas, and social media have seen them go viral (no pun intended).

Let us get back to some facts. One-third of Americans prefer to get news from the social media, 40% from Facebook. Fifty-seven per cent believe that social media news is accurate, and 42% have a great deal of trust in the media. A study from Associated Press showed that 60% of Americans get their information from the news, 40% go to official sources such as CDC and 30% listen to the daily press conference by President Trump. Approval ratings have gone up in April 2020: 44% of the population thinks that Trump is doing a good job, 29% thinks that the Congress is doing a good job, and 35% thinks that the country is going in the right direction (Betrus, 2020). Similar trends in trust have been found in other countries, although the trust in governments started to decline significantly in June 2020 (Fletcher et al., 2020).

I have conducted a scoping review of studies on traditional and social media during COVID-19, and their psychological impact (Vos, 2020a). This has led me to create the following formula:

Media misinformation + Exposure + Trust = Individual risk-perception

That is, the exposure to misinformation by the media that someone trusts seems to determine how they perceive their health risks (e.g. the risk of getting infected with COVID-19, of developing severe symptoms, and of dying from COVID-19). In the next chapter, we will see that the perception of health risks has significant consequences: risk-perception influences mental health and behaviour. Thus, we could formulate this fully, with the arrow meaning that the first part causes the second part:

Media misinformation + Exposure + Trust = Risk-perception → Mental health + Risk-behaviour

This chapter will explore this formula. We will examine the misinformation by media – with special attention for conspiracy theories – the role of exposure and trust, and how this influences our risk-perception, mental health, and behaviour. The last section will connect this media model with the political theories that we have discussed in Chapter 3: we may only understand the role of the media from its intertwining with political and economic powers. Throughout this chapter, it will become clear how the media use the uncertainties of the pandemic to sell their medium; they seem to bring stories full of the certainties that readers and viewers seem eager to pay for.

Table 4.1 Media model, descriptions and COVID-19 examples

Media model	Description	COVID-19 example
Misinformation & conspiracy theories	The general population seems to develop their perception, behaviour and mental health during pandemics on the basis of traditional and social media. Some information can be inaccurate, use logical fallacies, or include conspiracy theories.	Between 10% and 50% of information in traditional and social media seems inaccurate, including a wide range of logical fallacies and conspiracy theories.

(Continued)

Table 4.1 (Continued)

Media model	Description	COVID-19 example
Exposure & trust	The more individuals are exposed to news about the pandemic, and the more they trust the news source, the larger the impact will be of this news source on their perception, behaviour and mental health.	The amount of exposure and trust in the media predicts the perception, behaviour and mental health impact of the pandemic.
Political context	Traditional and social media sources can be influenced by their political and socio-economic context, such as their funders. Governments may manufacture public consent for their policies via the media and via other mind manipulation strategies. A critical attitude and critical education may help citizens to identify these influences on the media, and to determine their own perceptions and behaviours independently of the media.	There are some occasional stories about political influences on the media. However, more research is needed.

MISINFORMATION

Accuracy: Research suggests that in the first months of the pandemic, traditional media in many countries seemed to downplay the risks and severity (Betrus, 2020). In contrast, after the first weeks of the lockdown, news headlines suggested panic and outrage: 'Shambles, chaos, ridiculous' (*Guardian*, 1 April 2020). Subsequently, most traditional media have been underlining the risks and severity and have been supporting the nationwide lockdowns (Betrus, 2020). A scoping review and meta-analyses of 37 scientific studies on traditional and social media suggest that between 50% and 90% of all posts or news items about COVID-19 were in line with formal statements from the WHO, the national government or health authority, although these are very rough estimates (M = 69.5%, SD = 21%) (Vos, 2020a). These findings seem to be in line with studies about previous pandemics when news outlets misused statistics, exaggerated dangers, and even triggered xenophobia (Abeysinghe & White, 2010; Bird, 1996; Kilgo et al., 2018). During previous pandemics, the media seem to have contributed to widespread perceptions of large risks and anxiety by the high volume of coverage and an unbalanced emphasis on the threats (Klemm et al., 2016). During previous pandemics, a relatively similar percentage of 75% of all coverage was accurate, with inaccurate posts being shared more often on social media (Sharma et al., 2017; Tang et al., 2018).

Conspiracy theories: In the review of studies, several researchers also identified conspiracy theories (Vos, 2020a). It seems that during the COVID-19 pandemic, populism, and conspiracy theories – including the wide range of 'fake news' – are closely related, as many conspiracies involve the political and economic establishment. Let us now zoom in on conspiracy theories.

We may distinguish Conspiracy Theories – in capital letters – from conspiracy theories (Cassam, 2019). Everyone has some ideas which may be considered conspiracy theories by others. Conspiracy theories with small letters can be beneficial to states by stimulating transparency and democratic decision-making by those in power (Uscinski, 2020). Conspiracy Theories seem to be speculative, as they seem to follow from conjecture and educated guesswork, rather than knowledge and systematic solid evidence (Cassam, 2020). Conspiracy Theories often question issues of power, identity, and truth, by describing a small group of powerful individuals acting in secret for their benefit and against the common good (Uscinski, 2020). Conspiracy Theories often ignore Occam's Razor – also known as the parsimony principle – which says that the simplest explanation is the one most likely to be true, and are based on logical fallacies, as will be argued below (Uscinski, 2020). It has been argued that conspiracy theories should not be dismissed outright, but rather should be dismissed when the number of conspirators involved in the theory increases beyond the point at which secrecy could be maintained (Keeley, in Uscinski, 2020). Conspiracy Theories seem to become popular because they are 'first and foremost forms of political propaganda; they are political gambits whose real function is to promote a political agenda, and therefore they are not "just theories" like any other' (Cassam, 2020, p.7).

Stress and vulnerability: Under heightened stress and uncertain situations beyond one's control, people seem to lose their ability to weigh accurately and judge information (Brown et al., 2020; Fischhoff, 2012; Liston et al., 2009; Lerner, 2003). For example, the perception of a high risk of infection and mortality, deep anxiety and powerlessness correlate with the extent to which individuals believe in conspiracy theories (Allington et al., 2020; Biddlestone et al., 2020; Georgiou et al., 2020; Olesky et al., 2020; Sallam et al., 2020; Swami & Barron, 2020). This implies that we may not be able to discern reliable information from ambiguous or inaccurate information, mainly when the search engines and social algorithms prioritise content that seems to *align with our existing values and beliefs*. Often, the emotions that a news item triggers determine whether the item will go viral (Berger & Milkman, 2012). Fake news seems to reach more people and spread faster than the truth (Vosoughi et al., 2018). Conspiracy Theories can also go back much further in one's own life story. Often, Conspiracy Theories are a manifestation of socialisation, vulnerability, and a symptom of heightened danger from powerful actors (Uscinski & Parent, 2014). Research shows that Conspiracy Theorists are more likely to be male, unmarried, less educated, have lower household incomes, and see themselves as being of low social standing. They have lower levels of physical and psychological well-being and are more likely to meet the criteria of a psychiatric disorder (Cassam, 2019).

Cognitive biases: Logical fallacies are ways of reasoning that make an argument invalid and untrustworthy. I have asked friends and colleagues to send me some logical fallacies that they have observed regarding COVID-19. Table 5.2 summarises this. Research suggests that anyone can have logical fallacies in their reasoning and that this is not necessarily related to education level. Furthermore, although cognitive factors were significant in my COVID-19 survey, these effects could be explained by the feelings and existential interpretations of the health risks (Vos, 2020c). That is, although these cognitive factors are important, what ultimately determines the emotional impact and behaviour of individuals are their subjective feelings about their life in general.

Induction fallacy: The context of COVID-19 conspiracy theories is that two-thirds of Americans think that pharmaceutical companies spend less money on developing drugs that cure diseases because there is more money to be made by selling drugs that treat rather than cure diseases. Fifteen per cent also believe that new medical diseases are created to make money (Uscinski, 2020). Seen in this context, it is understandable that more than 20% of the population believe that COVID-19 is a hoax, 60% believe that the government is misleading them to some extent, and 10% are sure that China developed COVID-19 to destroy the West (NIHR Oxford Health Biomedical Research Centre, 22/05/2020). These are good examples of how empirical evidence can be blown up to gigantic proportions – which may be called induction bias. Chapter 2 has described cronyism and corruption by Big Pharma, and inappropriate influences on some decisions of international health organisations such as the WHO. However, there is no systematic evidence for a large-scale conspiracy; given the scale of the pandemic, it seems unlikely that this could have been kept a secret. Several researchers have provided good systematic and evidence-based debunking of common COVID-19 conspiracy theories (McLaughlin, 2020, https://www.kcl.ac.uk/).

Example 1: The pandemic was planned. Yes, scientists and charities have been warning about the advent of a pandemic like COVID-19 for decades, with the likelihood of it having increased due to globalisation and ecological collapse. They have concluded that governments and health services had not done enough to prepare themselves for a large-scale pandemic (see chapters 2 & 3). Scientists have been studying coronaviruses for a long time and therefore already knew much about how viruses like COVID-19 function and about how to develop PPE, treatments and vaccines. However, this does not mean that these researchers and politicians knew about a large conspiracy to cause a pandemic.

Example 2. Humans engineered the pandemic. There are many versions of this theory, such as China created the virus to destroy the West, Chinese spies stole it from a lab in Canada, or American soldiers brought it to Wuhan. US President Trump has fuelled some of these theories by claiming that China is responsible for the pandemic without giving any empirical evidence. Alternatively, some have claimed that Trump or his medical advisor Fauci are benefitting from the pandemic, for example because of Trump's financial investment in medical treatments. However, 11 independent research studies have shown that the virus's genome is 96% similar to a coronavirus found in bats, and the COVID-19 virus's spike proteins bind very tightly on human cells called ACE2 which may account for why COVID-19 is so contagious (Andersen et al., 2020; Xiao et al., 2020; Zhou et al., 2020).

Example 3. 5G causes or exacerbates COVID-19. Although 5G is higher on the non-ionising spectrum than 3G and 4G, 5G is not powerful enough to alter DNA, – lightbulbs would be more dangerous by this reasoning (*American Cancer Society*, 18/10/2020). Furthermore, despite the rise of exposure to radiation due to the widespread use of mobile phones, there is no evidence for an increase in brain tumours or cancers (Bensen et al., 2013; ICNIRP, 2009). Finally, 5G has also only been rolled out in a few countries, whereas COVID-19 can be found in almost all countries of the world.

EXPOSURE AND TRUST

We have seen how believing in conspiracy theories correlates with risk-perception and anxiety. However, it is difficult to discern whether the anxieties and perceptions of large risks make people read more about the conspiracy theories, or whether these theories make people more anxious and believe that they are at greater risk. Possibly, this could be a vicious cycle of media addiction, where people follow media because they are anxious and think there is a large risk, but the media makes them feel even more anxious and at risk:

Exposure → Anxiety + Perception of large risk → More exposure → More anxiety and perception of larger risk → etc.

Indeed, several studies indicate that the more time people spent on following the news or social media, the larger they perceive the risks to be and the more mental health problems they report (Ahmad et al., 2020; Gao et al., 2020; Tasnim et al., 2020; Zheng et al., 2020; Zhong et al., 2020). Thus, it seems the amount of exposure – or addiction – that precipitates the impact. Furthermore, other studies indicate that the media have a larger influence when people trust them, whereas individuals critical of the media will be less influenced in their perception and their mental health (Goodwin et al., 2020; Prati et al., 2011).

POLITICAL CONTEXT

If we make a logical jump and reason backwards from the research findings in the last section, we may argue that to improve mental health, individuals should limit their time on social media and news and should focus on news sources they trust. If health authorities want to get their message across, without creating mass panic, they may want to create a sense of trust, have one consistent channel of communication, and not induce too much fear. Thus, although governments tend to induce anxiety in their communications to motivate citizens to action, if fear becomes too great, this could become counterproductive, by shutting down the cognitive abilities of people to think and act rationally. Too much anxiety and too much coverage can lead to desensitisation, that is a diminished emotional response to news (Collinson et al., 2015).

Many scientific journals have published letters on the danger of misinformation, particularly on social media, during the COVID-19 pandemic. They refer to studies like those cited above, which show how the media have a substantial impact on how people perceive the pandemic and their adherence to precautionary measures. Therefore, it is not surprising that the social media giants

Facebook, Twitter and YouTube have started censoring information which they deem inaccurate. This censorship was usually conducted by algorithms specifically developed during the pandemic; consequently, errors seem to have been made by removing posts not containing fake news. Several people and posts were banned or deleted from social media, including Twitter campaigns from the US President Donald Trump.

Understandably, governments and the media seem to aim to create one consistent, evidence-based message by removing fake news, as this may hypothetically help in improving adherence to guidelines from the authorities. However, there are no studies on the effects of such large-scale censorship, which may be unethical when there are still so many uncertainties about the pandemic; there is not one clear truth and one logical way out of the pandemic. Looking at some trends on social media, particularly among Conspiracy Theorists, it seems that the censorship has created more mistrust of the media and politics. They argue that this censorship reeks of authoritarian governmentality. We also see this in research on risk-perception in the next chapter: people often create a distinction between what they recall about the communication by authorities and how they subjectively interpret the situation, for example by creating their own theories. The more mistrust is created by media and government – for example via censorship – the larger this gap will be, and thus the less effective will the communication from authorities be. In contrast, health authorities who recognise and address the emotions and subjective interpretations of the population, seem to be more effective in their communication (Sandman, 1987, 1993; Vos, 2011; Vaughan & Tinker, 2009). Thus, freedom of speech – and freedom of theorising – may be needed for the population to develop a relatively coherent perception and behaviour during a pandemic.

In recent years, a more critical attitude has emerged towards both traditional and social media. This is not only because younger generations are more internet-savvy, but people in general seem to have a more critical attitude towards the media (Campbell et al., 2006; Oliver et al., 2019; Westlund & Weibull, 2013). Several prominent books describe the relationship between politics and media. For example, the British author Owen Jones (2015) showed how there seems to be a revolving door between politicians, journalists, and large commercial companies. Ron Roberts and James Davies revealed some influences of pharmaceutical companies on how media portray mental health (Vos et al., 2019). Edward Herman and Noam Chomsky argued in their book *Manufacturing Consent* (2010, p.306) that mass communication media 'are effective and powerful ideological institutions that carry out a system-supportive propaganda function, by reliance on market forces, internalized assumptions, and self-censorship, and without overt coercion.' Herman and Chomsky argue that there are five filters which distort the news: size, ownership and profit orientation of the media; influence by advertisers; common sources of news have big powers; negative responses such as complaints and lawsuits by people who feel that their interests get harmed; use by politicians to support their wars such as the Cold War, the War on Terror – and possibly now the War Against COVID-19.

In my recent book, *The Economics of Meaning in Life*, I describe how the media are only one – although possibly the most influential – of multiple forms of 'mind manipulation' (Vos, 2020). Since the invent of neoliberalism in the Walter Lippmann Colloquium in 1938, economists and politicians have argued that politicians need to manipulate the minds of citizens to create support for their ideology. I have named this 'The Capitalist Life Syndrome', after the Stockholm Syndrome where hostages identify themselves with the hostage-takers. Neoliberalism seems to have been so successful in manufacturing consent in so many different ways, that many citizens seem unable to identify the socio-economic and political sources of what they regard as their meaning in life. My research has suggested that the dominant Western socio-economic-political system offers us unique perspectives on life, with a particular focus on materialism, hedonism, self-orientedness, and a functionalist or mechanistic approach to life and other people, and with a large impact on social, psychological and existential well-being. We grow up within these perspectives – we do not seem to know any better – and our perspectives get continuously reinforced by a society which seems to reward individuals with these perspectives and to punish those with alternative ideas. We seem to be seeing similar mechanisms during pandemics; in this and previous chapters, we have seen how people develop their perception, behaviour, and mental health of COVID-19 under the influence of their social, economic, and political context. From a critical-theoretical perspective, we may hypothesise that we may be experiencing a COVID-19 Life Syndrome, where public consent is manufactured via the media, biopolitics and lobbyists from the pharmaceutical industry. However, more evidence is needed to substantiate this.

HOW TO CREATE RESILIENT MEDIA COMMUNICATION

The best summary of the political and socio-economic context of the media was possibly given by Sue, a journalist who I interviewed for this book:

'Our editor-in-chief popped a bottle of champagne as celebration, when it became clear that the pandemic would hit our country. As he expected the pandemic to increase our readership – and he was right. But to get there, we had to deliver sensational stories.'

This chapter has shown how champagne-bottle-popping media moguls can influence our perception, behaviour, and mental health. We also saw that there is much misinformation in the media, possibly under the influence of politicians or the pharmaceutical industry. In times of scientific uncertainties, it seems unethical – and reflective of authoritarian governmentality – to be censoring opinions which deviate from the one message that the authorities want to convey. Censorship also seems ineffective: when media try to get rid of any uncertainties in the public messages via censorship, they could create a backlash, with more distrust of the public towards media and politicians. Therefore, authorities should guarantee freedom of speech – even if this means giving space to Conspiracy Theorists; the authorities will need to engage with the theories, as ignoring these could make them grow. More research and training in risk communication and media management is needed to prepare countries for future pandemics (Cooms, 2014; Glik, 2007; Ulmer, Sellnow & Seeger, 2017). Communication in times of scientific and governmental uncertainties such as pandemics is difficult, but it is possible when people trust the authority or news source. Trust determines how people remember, interpret and respond to public health messages, and thus trust can determine whether communications are successful in increasing motivation and intention to adopt or maintain recommended self-protective actions (Vaughan & Tinker, 2009).

Trust regards the public perception of the competence, fairness, honesty, caring, accountability, and transparency of the authorities. Health care authorities can stimulate trust by being transparent about their reasons behind action/inaction, timing, and errors in previous communications. Repeating messages and tailoring the message with clear instructions to specific vulnerable populations in outreach programmes can be beneficial. Research also shows how developing and implementing preparedness-plans could build public trust. There seems to be a clear consensus in the relevant literature and among experts that communication is most useful when this is open and transparent, and addresses the subjective interpretations, concerns, priorities, and culture of the targeted populations. Authorities should recognise and address popular interpretations and emotions – uncertainties, anxieties, and outrage (see, for example, Sandman, 1987, 1993; Calman & Curtis, 2010; Vaughan & Tinker, 2009).

An improved governmental communication strategy also means that governments should tailor communication to the targeted population. Usually, this implies, that theoretical explanation – or rational rebuttal of conspir-acy theories – is replaced with the simpler decision rules of heuristics and addresses the subjective interpre-tations and emotions (Reissman et al., 2006; Trumbo, 2002).

5

RISK-PERCEPTION

UNCERTAIN INTERPRETATIONS

'I know that the Prime Minister has stated that it is safe to visit stores, pubs and restaurants again. It does not feel safe yet to me, though. We are still at large risk to spread the virus and to become severely ill. Therefore I remain at home and order my grocery deliveries online. Ultimately, I feel that I know better what to do than the government.' (Interviewee Richard)

OVERVIEW OF RISK-PERCEPTION

Pandemics are extraordinary times for scientists and health authorities, as they need to make quick decisions while they still know relatively little. During the early stages of an infectious outbreak, there is often still much uncertainty. For example, at this time of writing, there are uncertainties about the precise number of people who could get infected with SARS-CoV-2 and who could progress to severe symptoms. There are no effective treatments or vaccinations available (yet), and the best government advice is to frequently wash our hands, keep physical distance from each other, and cover coughs and sneezes with a tissue – this is common sense, as this virus seems to spread via droplets in the air. However, it seems that only specific types of face-masks work in specific vulnerable groups, and that the overall enforcement of wearing any type of face-masks may not be effective. Using appropriate face-masks combined with physical distancing may only slightly reduce the infection rate in high-risk situations (Aggarwal & Dwarakanathan, 2020; Chu et al., 2020). Thus, it seems difficult to make hard conclusions that apply to each individual in each situation;

it is important to look at the risks of an individual in their context and the quality of the precautionary measures that they are taking. The only certainty that we have at this moment is that there is more uncertainty to come: pandemics rarely develop in perfectly linear and predictable ways.

Thus, health authorities are confronted with a devilish dilemma: while facing these scientific ambiguities, they do not want to risk the pandemic spiraling out of control and lacking health-care resources to treat those in need. Therefore, authorities need to act as early as possible, to prepare the health services for the worst-case scenario, and to stimulate citizens to take the appropriate actions, ranging from 'washing your hands more often for 20 seconds' to 'Stay at Home, Protect the NHS, Save Lives'. Although they may not be entirely sure about the best line of action, they often give stringent health guidelines: better safe than sorry.

This means that health authorities need to be experts in effectively communicating about risks, treatments, and prevention (Barry, 2009). They need to be able to give some clarity and certainty about the infection risks and the severity of the virus, – despite the unclear and uncertain science – and they need to clearly recommend or even enforce health behaviour that individual citizens could do to prevent the virus from spreading like wildfire in the population.

'In the face of an epidemic, terror, blame, rumours and conspiracy theories, distrust in authorities, and panic can take hold simultaneously. This is why establishing and maintaining trust through honest, clear communication is paramount. History continues to show us that health communication lies at the heart of epidemic control yet staffing for such communication is usually tacked onto health budgets as an afterthought, at woefully inadequate levels.' (Quick & Fryer, 2018, p.180)

When one person gives a message another person may receive this. The big question during pandemics is: will citizens understand the communication from the health authorities, and will they become convinced to behave in the safest way to prevent escalation of the pandemic? Will individuals change their habits?

However, there are often social and psychological filters between the sender and the receiver of information. Some information will get through to the receiver, but other information will not – metaphorically explained: like face-masks, filtering viral and bacterial particles. Researchers have called the psychological and social filters of citizens 'risk-perception'. To understand how people perceive and act during pandemics, we need to understand how they perceive risks. Therefore, this chapter will review the leading models of risk-perception, with examples of applications to COVID-19 (Table 5.1). This chapter will start with an exploration of our thoughts ('cognitions') and feelings ('affections') about risks. We will also examine how our risk-perception develops in social interaction with other people, culture, and media. Our perception is also embedded in the broader context of governmental strategies and global risks. Chapter 7 will add an existential risk-perception model, which will show how our perception is influenced by how we feel about the existential threat posed by the pandemic, and how we may still be able to live a meaningful and satisfying life despite this.

Table 5.1 Overview of types of risk-perceptions, descriptions and COVID-19 examples

Risk-perception model	Description	COVID-19 example
Individual risk-perception	Individuals may develop their own interpretations of health risks, regardless of what health authorities may have told them and what their recollections are of this communication.	Individual perceptions of risks associated with the COVID-19 pandemic seem to be relatively independent of the official communications by health authorities.
Social risk-perception	Individuals often develop their risk perception through social interaction, e.g. with friends, relatives, peers and the media. This social influence often depends on an individual's conformism, trust, disgust, need for social structure and outrage.	Individual risk perceptions are significantly influenced by traditional and social media.
Cultural risk-perception	Individuals develop their perceptions of pandemics on the basis of cultural values, e.g. about hygiene, which could function as ways to determine who is 'OK' and who is 'not-OK'.	There are examples of social exclusion/inclusion mechanisms.
Governmental risk-perception	Different governmental policies and communication strategies can have different effects on the perception, behaviour and mental health of citizens.	The amount of trust that individuals have in politicians determines the extent to which political policies and communication influences their perception and behaviour.
Global risk-perception	The lives of individuals are not merely influenced by their local, regional or national risks, but also by global risks and by international strategies to manage these risks. Health is a globalised phenomenon.	The pandemic started with a small outbreak in Wuhan in China, and has impacted almost all countries.

(Continued)

Table 5.1   (Continued)

Risk-perception model	Description	COVID-19 example
Unknown risks	Next to risks that may be calculated by scientists, pandemics seem to include many unknowns where a calculation of probabilities is not possible (yet). Individuals may find it more difficult to cope with unknowns than with calculated risks.	During different stages of the pandemic, there have been unknowns, e.g. about the severity, treatment and prevention of the disease.
Behavioural & mental health impact	Individual risk-perception is often an important predictor of individual health behaviour (such as using PPE, physical distancing and self-isolation), as well of the mental health impact of the pandemic.	Individual risk-perceptions significantly influence the behavioural and mental health impact of the pandemic.

INDIVIDUAL RISK-PERCEPTION MODEL

Most empirical studies on risk-perception have focused on the thoughts ('cognitions') that individuals have about health risks (Vos, 2011). Standard questions are, for example 'What is the likelihood that you will get infected by COVID-19?', 'What is the likelihood that if you get COVID-19 you may get severely ill?' Research participants could answer these questions with percentages or on a scale between 1, very unlikely, to 7, very likely. This enables researchers to examine how accurate their thoughts about risks are, that is: do their answers correlate with the formal communication by the health authorities? The underlying assumption of this line of questioning is that health authorities know the objective risks, even though, during the early stages of pandemics, they are often uncertain about this. These questions about rational thoughts are also very limited because the personal feelings and interpretations of risks seem to have a much larger impact on the psychological well-being and behaviour of individuals (Vos, 2011). It also appears that individuals distinguish their risks from the risks that others may have: others may be at great risk, but I may not be, and vice versa. Thus, more relevant questions than asking about mere rational thoughts are: 'How do you feel about your risk?' and 'Regardless of what you remember that health authorities have said, how do you interpret your personal risk?'

Remarkably, there have been few studies on the risk-perception of pandemics, even despite the importance of subjective perception to understand the psychological impact and behaviour of citizens. Leppin & Aro (2009) reviewed all studies on SARS and avian affluenza and found that researchers used a wide variety of risk-perception models to understand people's perception. Tooher and colleagues (2013) also found a small number of studies regarding the H1N1 flu pandemic. These reviews concluded that, although people are aware of the pandemic, they have a small to moderately accurate understanding of the health risks. Furthermore, their subjective perception of health risks was a much better predictor of their behaviour than the objective risks or government communication.

However, although many people intended precautionary behavioural actions, significantly fewer individuals engaged in preventive measures. I made similar conclusions when I examined risk-perception in other studies, which showed a gap between intention and behaviour: HIV, diabetes, cardiovascular disease, cancer, genetic counselling, vaccinations in general, smoking, safety at work, food safety and hurricanes (Brewer et al., 2007; Evangeli et al., 2016; Burnside et al., 2007; Hammond et al., 2007; Mearns & Flin, 1995; Nardi et al., 2020; Ndugwa & Berg-Beckhoff, 2015; Savasta, 2004; Slovic, 2001; Vernon, 1999; Warren et al., 2018). When I examined these studies, I found a remarkable difference between direct physical health risks and occupational/environmental health risks. The communication about physical health risks – such as cancer and cardiovascular disease – only had a weak influence on how individuals perceive the risks and almost did not influence their health behaviour at all; in contrast, official communication about professional and environmental risks had a much larger influence on people's risk-perception and behaviour.

This seems to suggest that people develop their own interpretation of relatively invisible risks such as pandemics, but they follow the communication of authorities more closely for risks at their work or risks from their environment. It is as if people reason 'I know my body best, nobody else can tell me what my risks are', whereas they may argue that they may not be an expert on risks at work or from the environment and in these cases they want to depend on experts. This was also what I found in my studies on the communication of health risks: although individuals may be able to have a relatively accurate recollection of what health authorities had communicated to them, they interpreted their subjectively lived health risks in their way, and their subsequent behaviour almost completely depended on their subjective interpretation and not on the officially communicated risks (Vos, 2011). Imagine this: a doctor tells you that your risk is 'A', you recall that the doctor said 'B', and you think that 'C' is really the case, but the risk feels like 'D', you do 'E', and you tell your relatives that their risk is 'F'. Elsewhere, I have compared this to a children's whisper game, where children sit in a circle and each child whispers a word to another, and there is no correlation at all between the word that the first child communicated and the word that the last child whispers (Vos et al., 2011).

How do these findings apply to COVID-19? I have conducted a systematic literature review of the risk-perception of COVID-19, and found an astonishing number of 123 studies – more than the sum of all studies on previous pandemics together (Vos, 2020b). Across all studies, I only found a weak relationship between either the objective risks or the governmental communication about the risks, and the individual's subjective perception of their risk of getting infected by COVID-19 and developing severe disease. Their protective behaviour is strongly predicted by their perceptions, but only to a small extent by their objective risks, as calculated for their situation based on the communication by health authorities at the time. For example, the government had communicated that there is a large risk of getting infected by COVID-19, but an individual felt that they were not really at high risk themselves and therefore they decided not to engage in rigid self-isolation. Alternatively, an individual felt that they were at extremely high risk – even though they were not in a vulnerable population – and they stuck strictly to all possible preventive behaviour, from frequent hand-washing to 24/7 self-isolation.

During this pandemic, I have also surveyed 562 participants (Vos, 2020, 2020c), and I found again evidence of the children's whisper's game model. There is a moderately strong correlation between government communication and an individual's recollection of this communication. However, their recollection is significantly different from what they think that their risks are, and these risks also feel differently for them. Subsequently, their precautionary behaviour is based on their feeling of risks, and not about their thoughts or recollections about risks. Thus, the children's whisper game strikes again! What individuals hear from health authorities is not how they feel about their risks, how they interpret the information, and how they act. Governments can communicate whatever they want, but ultimately this may only have small effects on their citizens' feelings, interpretations, and behaviour. This whisper-game phenomenon seems to apply across countries and cultures. However, when health authorities pay explicit attention to emotions, social interactions and people's underlying need for certainty, individuals may have feelings, interpretations, and behaviour that are closer to the health authorities (Sandman, 1987, 1993; Vos, 2011).

Why do people interpret health risks differently from what health authorities have communicated to them? Studies on previous pandemics have mainly focused on cognitive habits. The review from Taylor (2019) on pandemics suggested the following, which are in line with my previous conclusions (Vos, 2011). The more neurotic and prone to anxiety individuals are in general, the more they see health risks as personally threatening. The more difficult it is for individuals to deal with uncertainty in life ('intolerance of uncertainty'), the less accurate is their risk-perception, and the more they think that they are at high risk. Individuals who often search for information and scan frequently for health threats ('monitoring') seem to overinterpret their health risks compared to individuals who minimise or distract themselves from threatening information ('blunting'). Although some amount of optimism can be helpful to cope realistically with health threats, unrealistic optimism can lead to an underestimation of health risks. Some individuals also become very afraid when they confront any health risks ('health anxiety'), and their extreme emotional response seems to explain their overestimation of their health risks. Furthermore, individuals seem to overestimate their health risks when they misinterpret physical symptoms, interpret their current risks in the light of any previous diseases in their past, and focus their attention much on their body. Thus, these previous studies on health risks indicate that individuals seem to overinterpret their health risks due to general psychological problems or neuroticism, intolerance of uncertainty, health-risk monitoring, unrealistic optimism, health-anxiety, and narrow-minded interpretations and attention.

In my systematic review of 123 studies on COVID-19, I found a relatively similar pattern: the perception of COVID-19-related health risks depends on general neuroticism, monitoring or problem-focused coping, and optimism. Interestingly, numeracy skills, education level and intelligence did not appear as strong predictors of inaccurate interpretations and risk behaviour; our perceptions have more to do with our emotional, social, and existential processes than with rational reasoning.

> *'I know that I am not officially in the high-risk group. But I always seem to attract bad luck, and if anything goes wrong: it happens to me. Therefore, I feel that I am at high-risk, even though this may not be what the government or my GP would tell me. I do all precautionary measures as if it is very likely that I will get severely ill, and that I will die.'* (Interviewee Tom)

SOCIAL RISK-PERCEPTION MODEL

Individuals do not develop their subjective interpretation of their health risks entirely on their own. Often, people talk with friends and relatives and engage in whisper games where they tell each other thoughts and feelings which they subsequently shape in their subjective way (Vos, 2011). These conversations between non-specialists include gossip, personal theories and the collective memory of previous pandemics (Lupton, 2013). Risk-taking behaviour, such as not self-isolating when told to do so, seems to be influenced by the social norms that individuals and their friends have (Brady et al., 2016). My review of COVID-19 studies clearly showed how people's risk-perception and health behaviour were shaped by their social context and by social media. Researchers have argued that this social influence occurs via four social mechanisms.

Conformism: It appears that people easily conform to the ideas of friends, relatives, and colleagues and that they amplify each other's ideas. For example, one world-wide study of 7,000 individuals showed that in more than half of the countries, the individual's perception and behaviour were influenced by sharing individualistic worldviews, personal experience, prosocial values, and social amplification through friends and family. A good example is how peer pressure can influence individuals to get a vaccination (Cruwys et al., 2020).

Trust: Thousands of previous studies have shown how subjectively defining ourselves in terms of a particular social group membership affects our thoughts, feelings, perceptions, and behaviour (Haslam, 2014). For example, people feel that they can trust members of their group, even about topics such as transmitting risks of infections: friends, families and colleagues feel less risky than individuals from other groups, even though there is no rational argument to assume that they bear less risks. This implies, for example, that individuals may avoid close contact with strangers on the bus, on the street and in stores; in public spaces they may wear face-masks and gloves. However, when they are with friends or family, they may for example stay in proximity, shake hands, share drinks, or choose to visit one's ageing parents. People may also let go of their precautionary measures when they meet strangers with whom they share an identity or values, such as colleagues, or religious ideas.

Disgust: Several studies suggest that our bodies have a *behavioural immune system* (Schaller & Park, 2011). One definition tells that this is 'a collection of psychological mechanisms that enables individuals to detect pathogens in their environment and motivate behaviours that prevent these pathogens from entering the body' (Van Leeuwen & Petersen, 2018). This system usually works beyond our awareness and can respond to subtle cues such as strange smells or different looks. For example, people can feel disgusted about certain behaviours or specific people who are not in their social group; people are more likely to experience disgust in periods that they are more physically vulnerable to disease, for example during pregnancy. In contrast, people feel more comfortable being in a shared environment with ingroup members. These findings align with the evolutionary view that we are 'hardwired' to be more cautious of, or avoid, outgroup members because they are more likely to carry pathogens that we (ingroup members) are not immune to (ibid.). There are significant differences in how this system works in different people, as some individuals have a much more sensitive disgust alarm or feel more quickly frightened about their health than others (Taylor, 2019). However, this unconscious warning system often responds to superficial cues, which can result in a false alarm and aversive responses to situations and people who pose no actual threat of pathogen infection. This seems to explain why during pandemics, people seem very judgmental to others outside their group, which may even lead to xenophobia and other prejudices. An example of this in-group/out-group bias is how President Trump has frequently communicated via press conferences and Twitter about COVID-19 as 'the Chinese virus', and has been sketching other countries as dangerous while hailing the American approach to COVID-19 as 'tremendous'.

Need for social structure: A group of authors in social psychology has described how COVID-19 seems to have triggered mechanisms of thinking in terms of 'us' versus 'them' (Jetten et al., 2020). They show how our individual identity ('me') is embedded in our group identity ('us'), which can be differentiated from the identities of other groups ('they'). Consequently, our perceptions and behaviours are often influenced by others, social connections, collective behaviour, and relations with other groups. An example of in-group bias is an increased sense of national identity. Examples of out-group biases are some right-wing media such as Fox News frequently having cast COVID-19 as a 'left-wing hoax', and CNN which has criticised republican politicians – with President Trump at the forefront – to minimise health risks.

It seems that people do not like social ambivalence, and they are inclined to classify and structure the world in black-or-white terms, including specific individuals and excluding others. People experience acute discomfort and anxiety when they cannot classify the world: 'to classify is to give the world a structure: to manipulate its probabilities; to make some events more likely than others; to behave as if random events were not at random, and to limit or eliminate the randomness of events' (Bauman, 1990, p.1). Many empirical studies have shown that people believe in the meaningfulness and benevolence of the world and the explainability and control of events and that they will do anything to keep these assumptions intact, even during stressful times or after trauma; people will experience psychological stress when they are unable to develop a sense of meaning, benevolence, explanation and control (Janoff-Bulman, 2010).

However, this need for social structure is not only an individual process but also cultural: Bauman writes that this obsession with order is a typical task in modern times, an 'attempt to fend off chaos'. A consequence is that others may become 'degraded, suppressed, exiled' or pointed out as the cause of the virus, so that individuals and communities may restore their sense of trust and control in life, even though there is no conclusive evidence for the actual threat that others pose. Having an enemy has become constitutive of our own identity, regardless of whether the enemy are Democrats/Republicans, Whites/Blacks, Slaves/Slaveholders, Germans/Jews, Israelis/Palestinians, vaxxers/anti-vaxxers or maskers/anti-maskers. The political habit of living by the sword may feel like a new normal, but this may already have been our habit for a long time, albeit that this pandemic has made it more explicit (Mbembe, 2020). Full ethnic groups or nations have used this need for social structure, exclusion, and inclusion. Whereas groups or nations may lack a sense of meaning, identity or control, they could develop this by projecting their outrage onto others whom they may sketch as dark as possible, engaging in a war against the terror of their enemy. In contrast, the only real enemy may be themselves (psychoanalysts have called this process 'projection').

An example of social structuring is the black-or-white reasoning: 'you are safe' versus 'you are not safe'. For example, health-care workers have reported that they feel isolated and rejected due to the stigma of working with infected patients (Vos, 2020). Another example of the need for social structure is pandemic shaming. The term 'covidiot' was defined in the Urban Dictionary as: 'Someone who ignores the warnings regarding public health or safety.' Twitter shows, for example, countless pictures with the hashtag #covidiot. The British Health Secretary Matt Hancock branded people attending markets 'very selfish'. People may shame others because they feel insecure or anxious (Tangney & Dearing, 2003). Shaming can give a sense of connection in a time of social isolation: 'I belong to the group of heroes who will stop this pandemic.' Shaming can boost one's self-esteem – probably as a defence mechanism against feeling incompetent or ashamed themselves: 'Look how good I am!' Thus, publicly telling who is 'in' and who is 'out' can be the result of one's psychology. However, this inclusion/exclusion mechanism also seems to characterise modern politics, as will be elaborated in the next chapter. Additionally, the previous chapter has explained the role of traditional and social media.

Outrage: Peter Sandmans (1993, 1987) developed the controversial formula: 'Risk = Hazard + Outrage' (or more precisely said: risk is a function of hazard and outrage: $R = f (H,O)$). Experts often focus on the hazard, such as the infection and mortality rates of COVID-19, and they overlook the outrage. In contrast, the public often overlooks the hazard and focuses on the outrage, which Sandman defines as the strong justified emotion, for example, about the impact of quarantine and PPE on the daily lives of people. Whereas experts focused on reducing the hazard of the infection – for example via lockdown and PPE the public seems to focus on the impact of lockdown and PPE on their lives. This seems to be a good explanation of the protests and riots in several countries over government measures, such as the demonstrations by 'red-necks against face-masks'. Their COVID-19 outrage seems to be fed by what may be called 'the outrage industry' (Berry & Sobieraj, 2013). That is, outrage has become a genre of entertainment – with countless TV and radio shows with outraged hosts – newspapers, magazines and social media seem to sell via the outrage they express. Indeed, public outrage was reported during COVID-19 (Shananan et al., 2020; Trnka & Lorencova, 2020). In our 'age of anger', we see how individuals often respond with anger to stressful situations (Mishra, 2017). However, individuals could direct their outrage and anger at people other than those who have caused their frustration. Individuals could, for example, translate their experience of structural suffering and frustration due to socio-economic inequality and political disenfranchisement into anger towards innocent others, such as immigrants, instead of addressing the original political cause of their suffering (Milburn & Conrad, 1998). Research shows how frustration about the COVID-19 pandemic and the lockdown can translate into xenophobia, racism, and sinophobia (Devakumar et al., 2020; White, 2020). Sandman (1993, 1987) has advised authorities to explain better the importance of reducing the infection risks, acknowledge the public feelings of outrage and address the underlying causes explicitly.

'Yes, some people are at risk, and we should be careful with them. But the full lockdown is outrageous. They limit my liberties to live life to the fullest, and I feel that I do not have much time left to do so (as I am not the youngest person anymore), and now they even limit my opportunities more! I need people around me; I need others to feel OK. Therefore, I have been going to illegal parties every Friday during the lockdown. I do not understand people who take the lockdown too serious: what is wrong with them? During the lockdown I have learned who are "my people" and who are "not my people", often with unexpected findings, such as the biggest punks would be too afraid to go outdoors.' (Interviewee Sarah)

CULTURAL RISK-PERCEPTION MODEL

It appears that people often panic about invasions of their body by anything 'dirty' – unknown substances, microbes, or even symbolic experiences – consequently, individuals may start to protect the body from invaders and create a culture of 'Body McCarthyism' (Lupton, 2013). Marie Douglas (1986, 1966) has extensively written about the social and cultural construction of our perception and behaviour regarding hygiene and dirt. She shows how many cultures have their norms, values, and taboos about this, resulting in rituals such as Judaic hygiene laws, Muslim washing before prayer, and incense burning in Roman Catholic and Eastern Orthodox Churches. Some behaviour can foster health – for example the taboo against eating pigs was helpful for nomadic populations as the meat could quickly deteriorate in hot weather. Other behaviour can be less functional and more symbolic.

During COVID-19, the boundaries between functional and symbolic hygiene rules and taboos seem blurred. For example, although research is inconsistent about the effectiveness of wearing face-masks in public – at its best it has small or moderate effects on reducing transmission of the virus (who.int) – face-masks seem to have become *the* symbol of this pandemic. On the one hand, several governments oblige their citizens to wear face-masks, and studies suggest that many people indeed obey. On the other hand, in the United States, an anti-mask movement has emerged, where people break the taboos around self-isolation and personal protective equipment by protesting on the streets with placards saying that masks are an infringement of their freedom. This confrontation between 'maskers' and 'anti-maskers' does not seem to be about the actual functionality of face-masks, but about the social meaning. The symbolic character seems to be reflected in their referrals to morality: maskers call it immoral to go outside and not use PPE, whereas anti-maskers call it immoral to impose rules on people.

Marie Douglas (1986) shows how hygiene symbols and rituals can help us prevent personal and social collapse, and how uncertainties threaten the status quo. They define 'who is OK' and 'who is not OK', which group do I belong to and who is our enemy? She also showed that in response to risks, people often focus on strengthening the bonds and identity of their group, and how they define their heroes who will fight for freedom and responsibility. In general, in the confrontation with risk, society usually divides into four groups: hierarchalists who conform to the rules set by the authorities (e.g. 'maskers'); egalitarians who focus on the cohesion within their group (e.g. 'anti-maskers', people who blame outsiders, xenophobes, racists); individualists who determine their perception and behaviour; and fatalists who believe that their risks are determined by luck or fate. This seems closely applicable to our current pandemic.

GOVERNMENTAL RISK-PERCEPTION MODEL

As part of my review of 123 studies on risk-perception during COVID-19, I also examined the role of governmental communication, as we primarily learn about public health risks via public discourse, laws and institutions, albeit filtered by the media. Fifteen studies show that an individual's political perspective and trust in politics determine to what extent they believe the governmental communication and will follow their guidelines (e.g. Barrios & Hochberg, 2020; Dohle et al., 2020; Shao & Hao, 2020). For example, the more conservative someone's opinion is, the less they will follow governmental guidelines, whereas liberals are more inclined to follow the rules. With a similar variety of political opinions filtering risk-perception, the next chapter will describe the role of government in socially constructing the pandemic. This will show a variety of opinions, ranging from sociologists such as Giddens who seems to trust experts and, in their reflexive capacity, to philosophers such as Foucault who argued that modern governments set the norm with little reflexivity. They try to control citizens via policing or via making people feel personally responsible and guilty.

Based on countless studies, health authorities have recommended presenting health information in such a way that communication is perceived as credible. For example, research suggests that citizens will better adhere to governmental communication when they believe that: (1) the disease is severe and the recommended behaviours are effective in reducing these risks; (2) the person believes that they are susceptible to getting infected and developing a severe disease; (3) health authorities are regarded trustworthy; (4) it is easy to implement the recommended behaviour (Kanadiya & Sallar, 2011). Furthermore, citizens need to feel that the risk is personally relevant, that is the risk needs to feel very like their social group in their location in the present (Taylor, 2019).

There is also some research evidence from previous pandemics suggesting that people will adhere to government communication, when there is an emotional appeal in the communication, such as vivid descriptions of case examples (e.g. Slovic, 2001). However, evoking fear does not automatically lead to adherence, although this seems to be a general tactic in governmental communication during COVID-19. Fear induction without visualisation of examples and specific recommended steps is ineffective (Sandman, 1987, 1993). Individuals will adhere to fear-induced recommendations, when individuals perceive the threat as severe, see that they have the resources to give a good response, and believe in their capacity to respond appropriately (Peters et al., 2013). However, when communication is mainly dominated by fear, people may become hypervigilant for any health changes and may feel too overwhelmed to give a beneficial and proportionate response.

GLOBAL RISK-PERCEPTION MODEL

Several sociologists have argued that COVID-19 shows how much we live in a 'World Risk Society' (Sadati et al., 2020). Ulrich Beck (2009) coined this term to describe how we face many risks in our society, how we often think in terms of risks in our daily life, and how our risks are hyper-connected at a global level. We seem to see risks everywhere we go: while in the past going to a restaurant seemed to be just a non-reflected, joyful experience, individuals nowadays consider the risks, such as the use of ingredients that they may have a food intolerance for, the risk of food poisoning due to inadequate hygiene, the risk of going out in the wrong neighbourhood, and possibly even the risk of terrorist attacks. Our risks are also connected with others, even globally; for instance, scientists assume that bats caused the COVID-19 pandemic in the Hubei region, the virus was transmitted to animals in the wet market in Wuhan and spread globally via international flights.

However, we need to put the COVID-19 risks into a broader perspective. Our lives are always endowed with many risks. Objectively speaking, the individual risk of dying from COVID-19 is in most countries lower than the risk of dying from a heart attack or a stroke or in a road accident. Ironically, more people may die from the side effects and suicides triggered by COVID-19, than from COVID-19 (see next chapter). Why are we so obsessed with the risks of COVID-19?

Beck describes how globalisation has left out certain groups of people. For example, during COVID-19, not everyone has the right type of job, technological skills, and material resources to switch to online work. Manual labourers or those living on small budgets can feel that they are missing out and are outsiders in this increasingly globalised society. Others may feel that politicians have imposed a sense of cosmopolitism and multiculturalism, and the COVID-19 pandemics may seem to confirm their worldview that the world outside – e.g. Wuhan – is dangerous. Thus, COVID-19 seems to be the ultimate symbol of everything that is wrong with globalisation for anti-globalists. COVID-19 almost seems to have become an excuse to become nationalistic and close borders. Nationalism and provincialism emerge in response to global inequality. Therefore, it does not seem surprising that many conspiracy theories have emerged against symbols of this compulsory cosmopolitism, such as the WHO, or Gavi, The Vaccine Alliance, or global health charities such as the Bill and Melinda Gates Foundation.

The World Risk Society may also involve some forms of reflexivity. Individuals can look across their borders and see, for example, how other governments have dealt with COVID-19. They are also able to connect with people with similar values and interests anywhere in the world. In the World Risk Society, people are more likely to pose questions such as 'who am I?' and 'who do I want to be?' instead of automatically identifying oneself with categories pre-determined by their society. This seems to imply increased dissatisfaction and criticism towards one's government and scientists. Reflexive modernity involves the realisation that society may not be as utopian as people had imagined in the past (Beck et al., 1994). For example, the fact that experts frequently disagree becomes familiar terrain for almost everyone, causing laymen to join in the critical questioning of experts on everything including COVID-19: 'I know better than any medical experts.' In our hyperconnected online society, people can also quickly connect with others with similar fringe opinions, express their opinions and feel validated. Consequently, our era seems to be an era of outrage (see Chapter 5), as we have seen for example in the protests of self-identifying 'red necks' against face-masks in the US.

UNKNOWN RISKS

The previous sections describe risks that we know, or at least we know the likelihood that an event may happen. This does not mean that the event *will* happen, but it describes its likelihood. For example, smoking a packet of cigarettes a day for a long time significantly increases the likelihood of developing cancer and other chronic and life-threatening diseases; I may not develop cancer, but I know that by smoking I significantly increase my disease risk. Thus, risks bring the uncertainty of statistical probabilities, but I am more or less aware of the statistical likelihood and severity of the consequences. We know our risks, and we could do something to lower those risks, or prevent the event from happening at all. I could, for example, decide not to smoke.

Some researchers distinguish the following terms (I will not follow this distinction in this book, to keep the text simple): risk is about possible outcomes and their likelihoods which can be estimated; uncertainty is about possible clear outcomes with unknown probabilities; ignorance is about knowing neither probabilities nor outcomes; ambiguity is about a lack of agreement about the risks/outcomes/solutions (Stirling, 2008). Some researchers define Known Unknowns as uncertainties when we can neither estimate the probabilities nor the outcomes. We cannot control or manage these unknowns; the best we can do is to 'cope with the unknown'. Seen from this perspective, COVID-19 may confront us particularly with unknowns – more than risks – and probably because we are not used to coping with unknowns, as we usually frame the world and events in our lives consciously or unconsciously as statistical probabilities. We cannot see our blind spots, and suddenly COVID-19 confronts us with our blind spots. This may be one of the most stressful aspects of the pandemic: knowing that there may be something that we do not know and that we may not be able to control. However, many scientists and politicians seem to frame the unknowns of pandemics as knowns that we could control; however, these suggestions for control are not in line with Unknown Reality and give unrealistic power to people who have no power over unknowns. As we do not know what we do not know, we also cannot control what we do not know. For example, virus X may destroy humanity, and individuals may prevent X from becoming a pandemic by doing behaviour Y. As long as we do Y, we feel in control, and we can sleep well as we know that we did not do Y. However, when we know neither X nor Y, these unknowns seem to freak people out – just look at Hollywood movies about pandemics or zombie apocalypses caused by a small seemingly innocent incident like the bite of a sick monkey. Thus, people may respond in their daily lives to both the known statistical probabilities as well as the unknowns. The science of COVID-19 often seems to walk on this knife edge of known/unknown, and thus possibly plays with our ultimate fears of not-knowing; thus, we may release a sigh of relief when we hear the media presenting a pseudo-scientist or a populist politician who has found The Answer to Everything. Reality seems to be indeterminate – but we humans seem to want it to be determinate (Scoones & Stirling, 2020).

'Many messy, complex, open-ended dimensions of uncertainty are forced into a restrictive straight-jacket of "risk". Here, what are held to count as the relevant parameters are simply assumed to take a very few conveniently measurable forms. Values obtained on this basis for "probabilities" and "magnitudes" are presumed – as a matter of faith – to take the form of single precise, scalar numbers. And the results of all these highly subjectively situated procedures (often involving various forms of modelling) are then asserted as if they were precisely fixed "out there" in a supposedly objective world. None of these rhetorics of control are grounded in the more complex and intractable realities of uncertainty, but the resulting performance remains immune to the profound mismatch, because the pretence is so essential to organisational and political functioning. (…) Yet too often, risk is again instrumentalised, resulting in medicalised, securitised responses. This cannot address more complex disease ecologies, or how ill-health is generated through multiple, interacting factors, such as malnutrition, immunodeficiency

and marginalisation. Ill-health often emerges from structural inequalities, and is lived with, and experienced, by those exposed, generating often quite individualised emotions and bodily responses. In such cases, knowledge about outcomes is complex and indeterminate, and so not amenable to a conventional risk response. Instead, responses must be assembled locally by multiple actors (more than singular authorities), be constituted in social relations (more than categories of institutions), be rooted in context (more than universal standards) and deploy practical knowledges from diverse sources (more than elite disciplinary expertise). Effective responses to uncertainties around ill-health are therefore emergent, based on contestation and deliberation, and grounded in everyday practical and emotional experience.' (Scoones & Stirling, 2020, pp.12–13, 17)

BEHAVIOURAL AND MENTAL HEALTH IMPACT MODEL

We have seen how COVID-19 involves a combination of factors which make up an individual's perception of their health risks: individual, social, cultural, governmental, global and existential risk-perception. Whatever type of perception of health risks we focus on, the subjective perception is always a much stronger predictor of people's actual behaviour than the communication by scientists or governments. Like Sarah's perception was that the pandemic did not put her and her friends at a great risk of infection or mortality, and thus she decided to go to weekly parties. My statistical analyses of these studies showed that objective risks and government communication have a negligible influence on people's protective behaviour, such as using PPE in public spaces or self-isolating (naturally, these findings were corrected for enforced lockdowns when individuals were unable not to self-isolate). However, their protective behaviour was significantly predicted by their subjective risk-perception. This finding is in line with other studies that show how individual emotions predict their behaviour during pandemics, and how individuals can deliberately take risks, such as escaping the reality of the COVID-19 risks by going to large parties (Lupton, 2013). The next chapter will also show how one's subjective risk-perception is a crucial predictor of their level of psychological stress, anxiety and depression during COVID-19.

HOW TO CREATE RESILIENT RISK-PERCEPTION

This chapter has shown how people can relate to their body in multiple ways. We could metaphorically compare this with 'Body Worlds', the public exhibition of the inside of corpses. Although we may have relatively similar systems of muscles, nerves and bones, we do not look the same when we put our subjective experience on like our skin: we do not live in one world but in multiple worlds, as all of us have our unique perception and perspectives on the world. We are more than our biomedical facts, we have our own subjectively lived experience, which is shaped by our individual life experiences, social context and meaning in life.

How could our risk-perception become more resilient? Naturally, there is not one solution – one-size-may-not-fit-all – but health authorities could, for instance, more explicitly address the emotions, meanings and individual differences in their communications nationwide or to specific individuals (Vos, 2011). Health authorities could also more explicitly communicate how citizens could cope with self-isolation, such as reminding them of being physically active, actively reach out to friends and relatives, and engage in meaningful activities. Life experience could also help individuals to learn how to tolerate uncertainties and stress (Vos, 2016, 2011). Finally, educating people about the mechanisms of risk-perception and logical fallacies – such as reading this chapter – may help them to become aware of their own biases, and to make more conscious decisions about how to interpret and cope with adversity.

'The purpose of risk communication is to provide the public with the information they need to make well-informed decisions about appropriate actions to take to protect their health and safety. Risk communication should contain more than just tips about good hygiene and the need for vaccination. Ideally, risk communication should contain information about coping methods, strategies for dealing with stigma, guidance on managing stress when assuming new roles in the family, guidance on building resilience, and psycho-educational materials on grief, anxiety, depression, helplessness, apathy, frustration, anger and volatility.'
(Taylor, 2019, p.80)

Table 5.2 Common logical fallacies, with COVID-19 examples from social media

Logical fallacy	Description	COVID-19 example
Numbers don't lie fallacy	Arguing that we can trust numbers	The figures are going up, thus it is true that the pandemic is getting worse
Correlation is not causation fallacy	Arguing that because two phenomena occur at the same time, this must be true	Many death certificates say that people died with COVID-19, thus they must have died from COVID-19
Authority argument fallacy	Arguing that something is true because an authority has said this	The government knows best

Logical fallacy	Description	COVID-19 example
Slippery slope argument fallacy	Arguing that if event X were to occur, then event Y would (eventually) follow; thus, we cannot allow event X to happen	If we go to pubs and restaurants, a second wave may occur; therefore all pubs and restaurants must be shut down
Black-or-white thinking fallacy	Arguing that situations are either completely this or completely that	Either we go in complete lockdown or the pandemic will spiral down
Straw man argument fallacy	Arguing by creating a stereotype or inaccurate picture of an opponent's opinion, and attacking this false picture	People who go to restaurants are selfish
Statistical likelihood/fact fallacy	Arguing by conflating the likelihood based on statistical calculations that this must be true, ignoring that statistics often do not give a likelihood of 100% and often includes a variation around means	The scientific model was wrong because its prediction did not happen
Overestimating certainty fallacy	Arguing that a situation is more certain than it actually is, and dismissing any uncertainty	It is certain that the pandemic will be horrible
Bandwagon fallacy	Arguing that because many people think or behave in a certain way, this must be true	Most countries were in a lockdown, therefore Sweden should also have had a nationwide lockdown
Dunning-Kruger fallacy	Arguing in such a way, that the less you know about a topic the more confident you feel	I am not an epidemiologist, but I know what we should do
Cognitive dissonance reduction fallacy	Arguing in a way that removes any inconsistencies between thoughts, feelings and/or behaviour	The government has gone for a full-blown lockdown, and thus they need to come up with evidence to show how bad the pandemic is and to ignore counter-evidence and uncertainties
Emotional reasoning fallacy	Arguing on the basis of emotions	I feel that this is true
Availability bias fallacy	Arguing that because an example comes quick to mind, this must be generally the case	I remember having read in the newspaper about a case of COVID-19 in my neighbourhood, thus COVID-19 seems to impact many people here

(Continued)

Table 5.2 (Continued)

Logical fallacy	Description	COVID-19 example
Burden of proof fallacy	Arguing that because an argument has not been dismissed it must be true	I did not hear any counter-arguments, thus my opinion must be true
Worst-case scenario fallacy	Arguing that the worst case is likely to happen, and everything should be done to avoid this, even though there is no certain evidence that the worst will happen	This pandemic will affect everyone in society
Zero-risk fallacy	Arguing that no risks or negative cases can be accepted	We need to continue to be in a lockdown until there are no cases anymore
Fundamental attribution fallacy	Arguing that your own behaviour is due to your situation, whereas the behaviour of others is due to their personality	I cannot wear a face-mask because I am ill; it is selfish to see other people not wearing face-masks
Sunk-cost fallacy	Arguing that a course of action should be followed, even if the course has been found ineffective or costly	Because the government started the lockdowns, we must now continue with these
McNamara fallacy	Arguing by focusing on one specific type of figures and ignoring other factors	The number of COVID-19 infections are increasing, thus we must go into lockdown again, regardless of the psychological and economic side effects of the lockdown
False dilemma (There Is No Alternative) fallacy	Arguing that something must be the case because there is currently no alternative available	There is no alternative to bailing out the aviation sector
Self-serving fallacy	Arguing that one's own position is very positive, and dismissing other positions	I know best
Inductivist fallacy	Arguing by generalising a small number of cases	Based on the current COVID-19 figures, we must expect a second wave
Human impact fallacy	Arguing that humans can control everything	The virus must be man-made
Middle point fallacy	Arguing that a centre point must be true because the extremes at two sides of an argument get dismissed	There are both extremist right-wing politicians and left-wing politicians; therefore we must look for a solution in the middle

Logical fallacy	Description	COVID-19 example
Large conspiracy fallacy	Arguing that many people are in a large conspiracy together, ignoring that the likelihood of whistle-blowers becomes larger the more people are involved in a conspiracy	COVID-19 is created by the American and Chinese governments / The pandemic is all one big hoax
Common denominator fallacy	Arguing by focusing on the common denominator and denying variety	We are in this pandemic all together, thus black people should not ask for extra health-care
Falsifiability fallacy (related: cherry picking of evidence)	Arguing by looking only for evidence that confirms one's own argument, and dismissing counter-evidence	I have looked at the effects of the lockdown in the UK (and I ignored the effects of no lockdown in Sweden), and I conclude that lockdowns are effective
One-size-fits-all fallacy	Arguing that the same analysis or solution applies to all unique situations	All citizens in all countries should be in a lockdown
Is/ought fallacy	Arguing that from the situation that something is in, it can be derived how the situation should be	These are the numbers, therefore we must be in a lockdown
Idealisation fallacy	Arguing from the most idealistic outcome	When we find the vaccination, everything will be fine
Anecdotal evidence fallacy	Arguing by deriving conclusions based on a limited case	I know a COVID-19 patient who is getting worse, thus the pandemic is getting worse
Appealing to morality fallacy	Arguing by appealing to general morality	Do you not think that we should prevent people from dying? Therefore, you must go in self-isolation
***Post hoc ergo propter hoc* fallacy ('after this, therefore because of this')**	Arguing that because something did (not) happen, this must be caused by any prior events without giving further evidence for causality	The pandemic would have been worse if we hadn't been in a lockdown
Blaming the victim fallacy	Arguing that victims are to blame	If you had not gone out, you would not have been ill now

6

MENTAL HEALTH RISKS

UNCERTAIN MINDS

'Flattening the mental health curve is the next big coronavirus challenge.'
(Wong, 2020, p.1)

'Talking about how lockdown affects mental health doesn't make you a Covid-denier' (Jones, *The Guardian*, 13/10/2020)

OVERVIEW OF MODELS

'I am afraid of COVID-19. I am afraid of dying. Now I have also become afraid of living. I am stuck on my own in my tiny flat. I do not dare to go outside for a daily exercise. I do not dare to go to the stores. I do not dare to call my friends by phone. I do not dare to do a Zoom call with my family. What is going on with me? I know that I cannot get the virus via the phone or internet. I know that I do not fall in the group of physically vulnerable individuals. But still here I am, stuck in my life.'

Mary sighed deeply. I tried to look into her eyes which is always more challenging via the webcam than IRL. I saw the terror in her wide-open pupils. I felt sympathetic for her, as I could understand her feelings. I had seen the feelings of anxiety and being stuck in the review that I had done on hundreds of mental-health studies. I had read the answers in the Corona Survey that I had conducted. I had heard it in the interviews for this book. During our next psychotherapy sessions, I would try to normalise Mary's feelings: you are not crazy, as many others feel like you. I explained my research findings. I also asked questions about her expectations of life. How do you usually cope with uncertainty in life? How much certainty do you want? How much uncertainty do you have? How much certainty is realistic? What would it be like, to sit with this uncertainty, to look into its face, instead of running away? What would it be like to sit with the certainty of sickness and death, as everyone will get ill and die one day? What would it be like, if you were to start focusing on what can you do within the constraints of the uncertainties? What meaningful activities can you do? How can you make your house your home, full of meaning, for example by cleaning the place and putting pictures on the wall, instead of it being a prison?

After several weeks, Mary started going outside her house, visiting her family, and redecorating. She started connecting with others. She started connecting with her creativity by painting. And slowly, she started to accept the uncertainties of the COVID-19 lockdown, and she started to find new ways to live a meaningful and satisfying life despite its constraints. The uncertainties remained, but she had learned to live with them instead of fighting them.

This chapter will give an overview of the mental health impact of COVID-19. This impact seems to be frequently forgotten by governmental advisors and mathematical researchers, such as Ferguson. However, this chapter will show the importance of mental health. It will first give an overview of the mental health problems that people may experience, followed by an explanation of the different models of the causes of these problems (aetiology): models of organic causes, models of coping with stress, models of stress making one susceptible to infections, and models of the interactional-ecological and quarantine side effects. The following sections will describe how mental health problems may develop in stages and will highlight two common problems during pandemics: obsessive-compulsive behaviour and hoarding.

Table 6.1 Models of mental health, descriptions and COVID-19 examples

Mental health model	Description	COVID-19 example
Symptoms	Pandemics can have a significant impact on the levels of psychological stress and mental health of individuals.	Approximately one in two health-care workers report severe levels of stress or mental health problems, and one in three in the general population reports this. Patients with severe symptoms of COVID-19 requiring invasive medical treatment may report large long-term problems with their mental health.

(Continued)

Table 6.1   (Continued)

Mental health model	Description	COVID-19 example
Organic cause	Physical diseases may influence mental health, such as 'psychoses of influenza' and 'sickness behaviour'.	More research is needed to examine whether SARS-CoV-2 could be a biomedical cause of some mental health problems.
Stress-coping	The pandemic can have a different impact on different individuals due to the different perceptions and coping-styles of individuals.	The perception of high risks and frustration over the political/socio-economic situation has a large impact on mental health.
Stress makes susceptible	Individuals who experience large levels of psychological stress (for example due to their risk-perception or coping styles) may have a reduced functioning of their immune system, which could make them more susceptible to infections.	There are occasional reports of individuals with large levels of stress or mental health problems to be more susceptible to being infected and to develop more severe symptoms of COVID-19. More research is needed.
Interactional-ecological	Mental health can be determined by a combination and interaction of organic causes, perceptions, coping styles, stress levels and the political and socio-economic context.	There is some evidence that all components of the interactional-ecological model can explain the mental health impact of the pandemic.
Quarantine side effects	Self-isolation can impact physical and mental health via a combination and interaction of factors.	Some researchers have identified large numbers of excess deaths due to the side effects of the quarantine.
Stages	Individuals may experience different mental health problems at different moments of the pandemic. It can take significant time, and going through different stages of motivation, to change behaviour, thoughts and emotions.	Scientists have identified different stages in the mental health impact and in the motivations for change during the pandemic.
Obsessive-compulsive behaviour and hoarding	During pandemics, more individuals than usual may show symptoms of obsessive-compulsive behaviour and hoarding.	Reports across the globe confirm increased numbers of obsessive-compulsive behaviour and hoarding.

SYMPTOMS

Just before the COVID-19 pandemic got the world in its grip, we had been commemorating a centennial since the Spanish flu pandemic that had affected one-third of the world's population. In 1919, psychiatrist Karl Menninger had been working at Boston Psychopathic Hospital. However, the symptoms of his patients exceeded what was usually associated with the flu. In two papers, he wrote about 100 patients who experienced extreme mental disturbances, with a sort of psychosis in over half of them and hallucinations in almost two-thirds. Menninger was not the first to observe these 'psychoses of influenza'. After outbreaks of influenza in St Petersburg, Russia, in 1889, people had been reporting depression, suicidal thoughts, insomnia and homicidal urges during and after influenza (Honigsbaum, 2020).

Although the term 'psychoses of influenza' is no longer used nowadays, researchers have found psychotic symptoms in patients infected with SARS, and they have found an increased likelihood of individuals with schizophrenia to get infected with a coronavirus (Severance et al., 2011; Cheng et al., 2004). Other researchers have identified a so-called 'sickness behaviour syndrome' for people infected by a viral or bacterial agent (Dantzer et al., 2008). This includes symptoms such as nausea, fatigue, insomnia, depression, irritability, sweating, seizures, and problems with memory and attention. These are not merely responses to the fever but are different reactions to the infection (Corrard et al., 2017).

It has been argued that this sickness behaviour syndrome may explain some of the symptoms that some individuals experience long after the initial diagnosis of COVID-19 and even despite their negative test results. However, other causes may also underlie the symptoms that these individuals with so-called 'post-acute COVID-19 syndrome' (Greenhalgh et al., 2020) may suffer from, such as permanent organ damage to the lungs and heart, post-intensive-care-syndrome, post-viral fatigue syndrome and continued COVID-19 symptoms (*National Institute for Health Research,* 15/10/2020). Thus, there may be a wide array of interactional physical and psychological mechanisms underlying the symptoms of these so-called long-haulers.

In a systematic literature review and meta-analysis, I discovered 26 studies on the psychological impact of COVID-19 in 104,361 participants (Vos, 2020a). This showed that almost 60% of all health-care workers had reported symptoms of acute traumatic stress, and almost one-third experienced moderate to severe symptoms of depression, general distress, insomnia, or anxiety. One-third of all COVID-19 patients and the general population have also reported symptoms of anxiety, depression, stress and insomnia. I compared these studies on COVID-19 with 44 studies in 28,499 participants during the SARS and MERS pandemics. The impact of COVID-19 seems to be almost twice as large. One-third of all health-care workers and 15% of the general population experienced psychological symptoms. Then I focused on the most extreme cases when patients had suffered from acute respiratory distress syndrome or sepsis, or needed ventilation. One in two of these extreme cases reported severe post-traumatic stress, insomnia, and unemployment even years after hospital treatment (Chlan & Savik, 2011; Davydow et al., 2008; Davydow et al., 2013). Patients with severe symptoms of COVID-19 may experience similar long-term psychological effects. How worried should we be about these figures? We may argue that these mental health problems are a normal response to the abnormal situation of pandemics. The anxiety can even motivate people to take reasonable precautionary actions. However, the figures seem very large. In normal times, between 2% and 15% of the population report such symptoms, whereas 20% of health-care workers still report moderate to severe mental health problems several years after the SARS/MERS pandemic (Vos, 2020). Several studies have also reported waves of suicides at the end of pandemics, particularly at the two-thirds stage of the pandemic. Thus, COVID-19 seems to have a significant impact on mental health, and particularly on health-care workers – as it mentally impacted on Mary, who had been looking after her elderly neighbour.

ORGANIC DISEASE THEORY

Until the mid-20th century, psychiatrists saw a direct causal link between the infection and the mental health response. This hypothesis went out of fashion for a long time. However, more recent research has shown how sickness behaviour may be triggered by proinflammatory cytokines such as tumour necrosis factor-alpha, interleukin-6, and interleukin-1beta (Shattuck & Muehlenbein, 2016), and can be associated with neuroinflammation (Dantzer, 2009; Zhu et al., 2016). Other studies have suggested a significant correlation between influenza during pregnancy and schizophrenia in the child, albeit not very strong (Kępińska et al., 2020; Torrey et al., 1997). Other researchers have suggested that frequent infections and chronic exposure to infectious microbodies in our modern society could make individuals more vulnerable to developing stress-related mental health problems (Langgartner et al., 2019). These processes may explain the long-term symptoms of COVID-19, as one in five patients – particularly those with initially mild symptoms – have continued to have symptoms like the behavioural sickness syndrome (King's College, 2020).

However, more research is needed about the possible organic causes of mental health problems after influenza pandemics, specifically after COVID-19. These studies could have relevant implications as, for example, drugs for emotional disorders – such as antidepressants – may reduce the sickness syndrome (Dantzer et al., 2008).

STRESS-COPING MODEL

By the 1930s, the diagnosis of psychosis of influenza and its organic aetiology had gone out of fashion and had been replaced by psychoanalytic and behaviourist explanations. These models explain post-infection mental health problems as a result of failing to adapt psychologically to the stressful situation.

This new perspective could be explained by the stress-coping model (Folkman, 2011; Folkman & Lazarus, 1984), which hypothesises that when individuals perceive a situation as threatening and when they feel that they have insufficient resources to cope with this threat, they experience health-related psychological distress. This is where risk-perception comes in, as described in the previous chapter. Many studies on illness and risk-perception have confirmed, that the larger the factual health risks are, the more worried people are (Vos, 2011). My meta-analysis of studies showed that the more individuals interpret COVID-19 as a severe health threat to themselves and their loved ones, the larger the psychological impact is (see Chapter 2). For example, SARS-CoV-2 mainly puts older individuals and those with a chronic physical disease at large risk, and no vaccines or antibodies have been produced yet to prevent or treat COVID-19. Due to this considerable health risk and lack of resources to prevent or treat it, these individuals worry more and suffer from more psychological distress, anxiety, and depression. Furthermore, an updated version of the stress-coping model shows that meaning in life can be an essential buffer in coping with stress. Having a sense of meaning in life is, for example, associated with better functioning of the immune system and other biomarkers (Vos, 2016). Chapter 8 will elaborate on the existential coping process with stressful life situations such as the COVID-19 pandemic. A good example is how Mary perceived that she was at great risk and that she could transmit this risk to her vulnerable elderly neighbour who she was looking after; in response to her fear, she decided to stay inside, as she felt that she did not have the resources to continue doing what she was doing, including helping the neighbour; she felt that the only opportunity was staying inside her flat.

In my Corona Survey, I also examined the relationship between risk-perception and the level of mental health problems (MHP – measured as anxiety, depression, and general psychological stress in structural equation models). I found the following: the recollection of governmental communication about the COVID-19 risks has a small to moderately strong impact on MHP. Instead, their subjective interpretation of these risks strongly predicts their MHP. Thus, their mental health strongly depends on their subjective interpretation of the pandemic risks and not on what governments communicate. Their MHP was also strongly predicted by their subjective interpretation of the severity of COVID-19, the trust in treatment options, and the trust in preventive measures; in contrast, their recollection of the governmental communications did not predict MHP. Furthermore, individuals who were objectively at a higher risk of infection or severe symptoms – such as individuals over 70 years or those with underlying diseases – accurately recalled they were at greater risk, and their recollections had a moderately strong effect on their MHP; however, like others, their subjective interpretation had a strong impact on MHP. Their recollections of the formally communicated risks did not correlate with their subjective interpretation of these risks, and they were also significantly different from each other. When I looked at the intention to use PPE and to self-isolate, these intentions were to a small extent predicted by their recollections of the government communication and to a large extent by their subjective interpretations. In sum, people seem to make a subjective difference between what governments tell us about the risks of COVID-19 and how they interpret these risks themselves. What matters for their mental health and their behaviour are mainly their subjective interpretations. These findings are in line with previous studies on the impact of risk-perception on MHP and health behaviour (Vos, 2011). Thus, these findings indicate that the stress-coping model may be a good explanation of MHP during pandemics.

STRESS MAKES INDIVIDUALS SUSCEPTIBLE TO INFECTIONS MODEL

We have discussed how both organic and psychological mechanisms could lead to mental health problems. However, decades of research have also shown how psychological stress and mental health problems could make individuals more susceptible to infections. For instance, there are occasional reports of psychiatric patients having a greater likelihood of getting infected with SARS-CoV-2 (Xiang et al., 2020; Yao et al., 2020). Furthermore, stress is associated with an increased susceptibility to upper respiratory infections and common colds (Pederson et al., 2010; Cohen et al., 1991). Stress seems to lead to this greater susceptibility to infection due to the influence of stress on the production of lymphocytes and proinflammatory cytokines (Freestone et al., 2008; Glaser & Kiecolt-Glaser, 2005; Yang & Glaser, 2000; Cohen, 1996). Several studies show that the experience of acute psychological stress after a trauma leads to poorer general physical health and mortality in the short and long term (Garfin et al., 2018). The beneficial effects of vaccines can also be substantially reduced due to stress, particularly among individuals with frequent negative moods (Phillips et al., 2005; Glaser & Kiecolt-Glaser, 2005). Thus, there seems to be strong evidence that psychological stress and mental health problems could make people more susceptible to infections and other physical health problems. However, more research is needed to examine whether psychological therapies could also improve the functioning of the immune system and the susceptibility to infections (Moraes et al., 2018).

INTERACTIONAL-ECOLOGICAL MODEL

Whereas in the past researchers seemed to say either 'everything is in the mind' or 'everything is in the body', nowadays many think in terms of complex systems (Vos et al., 2019). Body and mind often interact. Furthermore, this interaction also needs to be seen in synergy with the social context, as socioeconomic inequality is associated with more psychological stress and increased susceptibility to diseases (see previous chapter). Thus, physical, psychological, and socio-economic health seem to be intertwined.

Let us return to the meta-analyses of mental health studies on COVID-19, SARS, and MERS. I looked at the causal factors identified in these studies (Vos, 2020). The findings suggest a complex interaction of factors, with a strong focus on the psychological impact of the socio-economic and political context. I found that health-care workers suffer from more mental health problems when they feel dissatisfied with the organisation, training, and support at work, as well as the lack of personal protective equipment and funds allocated by the government. They also report more stress due to a lack of social support from colleagues, friends, and family, and when they are in direct contact with infected patients. In the general population, individuals experienced more psychological problems when they belonged to a physically or mentally vulnerable population, such as having an underlying physical disease or being older – which makes sense. Furthermore, individuals with low socio-economic status experienced more psychological problems. The lockdown also increased mental health problems, with half of the isolated individuals having acute post-traumatic stress disorder or depression. A large part of the psychological impact of pandemics is caused by political decisions that involve a lack of adequate equipment, inefficient health-care organisation, long-term nationwide lockdown, and socio-economic inequality. Thus, COVID-19 seems to impact our mental health due to a combination of physical, psychological, and socio-economic factors.

QUARANTINE SIDE EFFECTS

In Ancient Greek, the word 'pharmakon' meant both cure and poison. Similarly, Esposito (2020) wrote that in modern societies, the poison of suffering or death could be imposed on individuals for the greater good of the abstract concept of bare Biological Life (Agamben, 2020). Similarly, politicians seem to justify nationwide lockdowns by referring to stopping the spread of the virus and dismissing the harm to specific individuals. Our meta-analyses of COVID-19 studies found that physical isolation, either nationwide lockdown or self-isolation, is associated with symptoms of post-traumatic stress, depression, and insomnia (Vos, 2020). Interview studies on the impact of quarantine during previous pandemics had similar conclusions (Brooks et al., 2020).

A review of 24 studies on the impact of quarantine during COVID-19 also suggested a large short-term psychological impact, although the reviewers argued that these psychological side effects may be small compared to the effects on reducing the infection rates (Vali et al., 2020). Similarly, a systematic review of 51 studies suggests that the temporary or partial implementation of quarantine early on in a pandemic and combining quarantine with other public health measures such as physical distancing, can help slow the spread of COVID-19 (Cochrane, 29/09/2020). However, these studies did not compare the short-term impact of quarantine on the infection rates with the long-term physical and mental impact of the lockdown, such as missed appointments due to closed hospitals and suicides. Furthermore, although 92% of the British population support quarantine, 44% report that they suffer significantly due to quarantine (Jetten et al., 2020).

Thus, although large-scale lockdowns and quarantines may help to limit the spread of the virus in the short term, these can also have a large negative impact on the long-term. Several mechanisms seem to explain these negative side effects of lockdowns and quarantines.

First, individuals in quarantine are less physically active, although research suggests that physical inactivity can worsen mental well-being (Bauman, 2004; Hoare et al., 2016; Penedo & Dahn, 2005). Second, individuals miss the daily routine, which could have an impact on their sleep/wake patterns and subsequently their mood (Shananan et al., 2020). Third, isolated individuals feel bored and engage less in leisure activities (Marafa & Tung, 2004), which could minimise the opportunities to release psychological and physical stress (Aldana et al., 1996; Weng & Chiang, 2014). Fourth, people have less social contact, mainly with single or stigmatised individuals Best et al., 2014; Jeong et al., 2016). However, research shows that social contact has a strong positive effect on mental health (Hawkley & Caccioppo, 2010; Heinrich & Gullone, 2006; Holt-Lunstad et al., 2015; Mushtaq et al., 2014). Fifth, individuals may have financial worries and feel stressed over unemployment or housing (Atkeson, 2020; Jeong et al., 2016; Stephany et al., 2020; Yilmazkuday, 2020). Sixth, large families may experience more stress due to the emotional impact on children and family interactions (Brooks et al., 2020; Grechyna, 2020; Liu et al., 2020). Seventh, inadequate supplies may lead to a deterioration in people's dietary and health behaviour, which could also impact on their emotional well-being (Jeong et al., 2016). Eighth, quarantine could lead to more psychological stress, and we have seen how stress can lead to reduced immune system functioning and greater infection risk (Biondi & Zannino, 1997; Garfin et al., 2018; Segerstrom & Miller, 2004). Ninth, self-isolation can also lead to suicides – extrapolating from previous pandemics, we may expect approximately 200,000 deaths worldwide during the COVID-19 pandemic. What these studies seem to have in common is that they describe how people struggle to live a meaningful and satisfying daily life within the constraints of quarantine (Pereira et al., 2020; Tabri et al., 2020; Vos, 2020). Tenth, research from several British governmental bodies have indicated that for every three deaths caused by a coronavirus, there were another two caused by the impact of the lockdown (DHSC et al., 2020). The nationwide lockdown may have indirectly caused 8,000 excess deaths per month in the UK. They mainly attribute this to a reluctance to attend A&E or GP surgeries and having difficulties accessing medical assistance as all non-urgent medical appointments had been cancelled. They also estimate an increase of 18,000 excess deaths in the longer term as a result of the lockdown-induced recession. Thus, their research did not include any of the other psychological variables reported above, and thus their numbers may be on the low side.

In sum, may the cure be worse than the disease? Mary was still doing relatively well from a mental health perspective, but merely staying inside seemed to have caught her in a spiral of negative emotions. The decisive mathematical models from researchers such as Ferguson did not take these psychological and social side effects into account when they recommended nationwide lockdowns. However, there may not be one perfect strategy, as not having a lockdown may have led to a larger spread of the virus: there is clear evidence that a lockdown early during the pandemic has significantly slowed down the number of COVID-19 infections (Garikipati & Kambhampati, 2020; Lau et al., 2020). The governmental report also suggested that the lockdown may have prevented an escalation of the pandemic (DHSC et al., 2020). However, the science on lockdowns is ultimately limited by many uncertainties, as there are few systematic studies on this complex dynamic phenomenon. Therefore, multidisciplinary teams of experts – including ethicists – will need to identify for each pandemic in each unique location at each unique time what is the least-worst option.

STAGES

Our emotions rarely remain the same – our emotional life changes in response to changing circumstances and our change perceptions of these. For example, Bechtel and Berning (1990) observed that individuals mainly report psychological stress during the third quarter of fixed-term situations of isolation and stress. Reports on suicide rates during pandemics seem to indicate a similar trend: when the pandemic is almost over, there seems to be a spike in the number of individuals taking their own lives (Vos, 2020). Over the years, psychologists have developed many models to explain the stages in the emotional adjustment to stressful life circumstances, some of which I will now introduce.

Try to remember when you heard about the first cases of COVID-19. Try to remember when you heard that you had to go into a lockdown. Try to remember a stressful moment during the pandemic. Most likely, the first response when you learned about the stressful situation was one of alarm or shock. The body acts as though it is injured, by lowering blood pressure and body temperature. After this, your sympathetic nervous system gets activated, pumping adrenalin through your body, preparing you to either fight, flight, freeze or feed. After a while, your body may seem normal again, but the stress hormone cortisol is released and unnecessary body functions are shut down. When you remain in a stressful situation for a long term, your physical resources may become depleted, your immune system could become weakened, and the prolonged release of adrenalin can have adverse effects on the body, leaving it susceptible to illness and disease. This is a summary of the General Adaptation Model to Stress (Selye, 1950). Most individuals will not have encountered situations which triggered extreme stress responses, as they did not perceive the stressors as very threatening or that they had sufficient resources to deal with these (Vos, 2016). However, in my Corona Survey, individuals reported that they experienced higher levels of psychological stress and more physical symptoms indicative of a reduced immune system when they perceived the infection and mortality risks of themselves and their loved ones as large (Vos, 2020b). Even relatively low levels of psychological stress seem to reduce immune system function in the long term, as it may deplete bodily resources. Thus, the more afraid you are of getting COVID-19, the worse your immune system functions, and hypothetically the more susceptible you are to infections.

Several psychological pop-science magazines have explained the grief model of Kubler-Ross during the pandemic. Authors argued that people might not only be mourning over the loss of a loved one, but they may also be grieving over the loss of their old life and struggling with the emergence of a 'new normal'. Kubler-Ross has described how individuals could experience grief in the stages of denial, anger, bargaining, depression, and acceptance. Although many individuals recognise that they experience different emotions at different points in time, research shows that these emotions often do not follow a linear path and multiple emotions could happen at the same time (Stroebe et al., 2017).

Another staging model has frequently been cited during the pandemic: the Transtheoretical Model, also known as the Stages of Change Model. This model describes the stages of change that individuals may go through when they consider making life changes, such as frequent hand-washing, using a mouth mask or physical distancing. Stage 1 of behaviour change is about precontemplation, when people are not considering a change, and instead are denying that they may need to change their behaviour, or they are avoiding any news or reminders of the pandemic. Stage 2 consists of increased awareness of the potential benefits of behavioural changes, but often individuals experience uncertainty, ambivalence, and conflicted emotions, and they do not know how to overcome practical barriers to change. In stage 3, individuals start experimenting with some small changes, and collect information about what to do, or get support from others. In stage 4, people take direct action to accomplish their goals. Stage 5 consists of the maintenance of the 'new normal' and avoiding temptations to return to old habits. Some individuals – but not all – may have a temporary or permanent relapse (stage 6), such as forgetting to use PPE or being fed up with physical distancing and not meeting friends and relatives; this relapse could make them feel disappointed or frustrated about themselves. Several studies have suggested that individuals can indeed go through these stages of change during COVID-19, although often these steps are not totally linear, and individuals could fall back or skip a stage. Health authorities could use this model to structure their communications, and to develop interventions for at-risk individuals (Faulkner et al., 2020; Hoti et al., 2020; Noori, 2020; Romano, 2020; Xu et al., 2020).

Thus, we see that psychological progress is not as linear as we may expect, but instead, it is often gradual, messy, and circular. Life does not seem to fit into our idea of linear progress – going in a straight line from the starting point, via several stages, to our goal. This idea of linear progress seems typical of modern science and seems to have mainly evolved in capitalist countries during recent centuries (Vos, 2020). We seem lost when we cannot identify the precise start and end of our experiences. Not knowing the stages or 'the roadmap' of the pandemic seems to frustrate and frighten people (see Chapter 1).

In contrast, less capitalist and ancient cultures seem to focus more on the idea of gradual change and circularity – like the change of the seasons, the death and rising of the Phoenix, and the Hindu god Ganesha who simultaneously symbolises endings and new beginnings (Vos, 2020, 2018). Our subjectively lived experience of life often seems more in line with these pre-modern concepts (Vos, 2005). Our societies now seem to be in a moment of transition, between our pre-COVID-19 life when we thought we knew where we were and where we were going in life, and our unknown future living with our COVID-19 experience. Our past is not completely there anymore, and the future is not completely there yet; we are confronted with a double nothing-ness, being-in-limbo, that seems to be psychologically stressful and existentially frightening (see next chapter). Pre-modern cultures and religions, such as Hinduism and Buddhism, recommend staying with our experiences of uncertainty and nothingness, instead of pushing these away with our imperfect explanations and models. Buddhism tells that suffering arises from our tendency to push away our experiences of reality with our thoughts, explanations, and models. Instead, the Buddha suggests learning to tolerate uncertainties, sitting with both our positive and negative experiences instead of running away, and taking each moment as it reveals itself while recognising and actively using the small opportunities to take control and understand these parts of our daily life (Vos, 2020).

OBSESSIVE-COMPULSIVE BEHAVIOUR AND HOARDING

Two types of rigid behaviour have attracted much attention during the pandemic: obsessive-compulsive behaviour and hoarding (Banerjee, 2020).

For example, Mary had hoarded many piles of toilet paper rolls and canned food, and she would only order food deliveries online, the boxes of which had to be left outside her door so that she did not need to have any contact with the delivery people.

Obsessive-compulsive behaviour is the experience of frequent obsessive thoughts and compulsive behaviours (nhs.org.uk). An obsession is an unwanted and unpleasant thought, image or urge that repeatedly enters the mind, causing feelings of anxiety, disgust, or unease. A compulsion is a repetitive behaviour or mental act that someone feels they need to do to temporarily relieve the unpleasant feelings brought on by the obsessive thought. For example, an individual can be terrified of getting infected and therefore continuously washes their hands – for more than 20 seconds, and even after recently washing – and rigidly stays indoors at home. If they need to go outside they will take many precautions, possibly not just wearing a simple face-mask but a high-quality gas-mask, gloves or even a laboratory suit. Of course, this is a sliding scale, as some obsessions and compulsions are reasonable and have been prescribed by health authorities to minimise infection risks. However, obsessive-compulsive behaviour could become so rigid and extreme that it goes beyond the cultural norm, that the person has lost control over it, and that it limits the individual in their social and professional life.

It is easy to see how the recommendations in the media for 'proper' hand-washing steps, PPE and physical isolation can stimulate obsessive-compulsive behaviour, particularly in individuals who have had similar symptoms or were prone to anxiety before the pandemic. Often, obsessive-compulsive behaviour is the result of negative subjective interpretations and exaggerations of governmental communication. This perception of extreme risks leads to physical reactions such as hyper-arousal and hyper-vigilance. This could, for example, make an individual jump with anxiety when they enter a situation or experience a reminder of their feared scenario – such as seeing an individual without a face-mask coughing in a public space. By not going outside and not exposing themselves to the feared scenario, people feel that they control their anxiety; they prevent confrontation with the feared scenario. However, compulsive behaviour could become a habit – 'it feels right' – to stay at home and engage in rigid precautionary behaviour. This habit of avoiding confrontation with their fear could generalise to other situations, such as avoiding low-risk daily-life situations, and thus this habit could raise the threshold to return to daily life after the pandemic. (This paragraph is based on cognitive-behavioural models: see Clark, 2004; Salkovskis et al., 1998.)

The hoarding of toilet paper, hand sanitiser, face-masks and canned food is possibly one of the most iconic symbols of the COVID-19 pandemic. Globally, shops ended up with empty shelves for weeks or months, due to customer stockpiling (Oosterhoff, 2020). Naturally, it was rational to buy protective equipment and food rations in case one became ill and not be able to go to the stores. However, the extent to which stores were completely emptied seems beyond reason.

A hoarding disorder is where someone acquires an excessive number of items and stores them in a chaotic manner, usually resulting in unmanageable amounts of clutter (nhs.org.uk). Hoarding is considered a significant problem if: the amount of clutter interferes with everyday living, or the clutter is causing significant distress or negatively affecting the quality of life of the person or their family. Hoarding seems to be associated with risk-perception: the larger the infection risk is in one's subjective interpretation, the more likely will individuals buy goods that no longer follow common sense (Garbe et al., 2020; Long & Khoi, 2020). Behavioural economists have also shown how the idea of scarcity can lead to hoarding: the more individuals become afraid that essential items will run out, the more likely it is that they will buy these products. People are afraid that they will miss out. Ironically, due to their fear of scarcity, they create the scarcity that they fear (Baddeley, 2020; Kirk & Rifkin, 2020). Thus, anticipatory anxieties and emotionality seem to underlie panic buying and hoarding (Arafat et al., 2020; Garbe et al., 2020). COVID-19 can remind people of their mortality, which could lead to an increase in spending to offset fear (Arndt et al., 2004). That is, consumer goods are more than functional: brands and products can make us feel good, and this positive feeling can push aside our fears of illness and mortality. This so-called 'Terror Management Hypothesis' will be elaborated in Chapter 7. Thus, these results seem to emphasise the importance of clear communication by public authorities acknowledging anxiety and, at the same time, transmitting a sense of control (Garbe et al., 2020).

HOW TO CREATE RESILIENT MENTAL HEALTH

When a disaster happens in movies, we often see chaos and people acting illogically or in unreasonable ways. However, the reality is different. Most research shows that such a disaster syndrome does not exist and that people hold onto the tenets of acceptable behaviour, such as following the law and morality (Savage, 2019; O'Leary, 2011). However, this is not to say that people are not suffering – as this chapter has shown, pandemics, and particularly working at the front line or being in quarantine, can have a large impact on our mental health.

How could we improve mental health? Table 6.2 gives examples of how individuals could improve their psychological well-being, particularly during lockdown. Table 6.3 gives recommendations for health-care policy-makers (see also Ornell et al., 2020). When these preventive and self-helping strategies are not sufficient to maintain good mental health, psychological therapies and counselling may be beneficial. At the time of writing, there are approximately 11,000 publications on mental health-care during COVID-19. Specifically for this chapter, I have conducted a scoping review and meta-analysis of 67 clinical trials that had one measurement before the first session and one after the last session. Regardless of the type of client and the type of psychological help, the psychological treatment had brought about large improvements in the most common mental health problems of anxiety and depression (Hedges' g = 0.83, SE = 0.31, p < 0.001). The effects of individuals with high levels of anxiety and depression were larger than on those with moderate or small levels (Cohen's d = 0.35, p < 0.01).

It is beyond the scope of this book to advise on how mental health-care professionals can help individuals. However, in line with the existential nature of the pandemic, a humanistic or existential approach in psychotherapy – as with my work with Mary (Serlin & Cannon, 2004) – may be recommended. During collective disasters and grief, people can benefit from reconstructing their perception of the world and meaning in life (Schulenberg et al., 2014; Neimeyer, 2001). This means that therapists explicitly address the existential challenges of the pandemic and help clients to find ways to live a meaningful and satisfying life despite these challenges (Vos, 2018). Reviews show that such existential and meaning-oriented therapies can be particularly effective in individuals struggling with health, health risks and existential threats (Vos & Vitali, 2018; Vos et al., 2014).

Table 6.2 Recommendations to individuals for maintaining individual mental health (based on MentalHealth4All.org)

Recommendations
Keep in touch with friends and family, e.g. via email, phone, or video conferencing
Keep a daily routine and sleep pattern
Make time for leisure, relaxation, and laughter
When possible go into nature, e.g. for a walk in a park
Do physical exercises, inside or outdoors

(Continued)

Table 6.2   (Continued)

Recommendations

Make your house your home, e.g. clean and put meaningful pictures on the wall

Limit exposure to pandemic-related and frightening news

Follow the advice from official health authorities, e.g. WHO, CDC, NHS

Pay attention to your needs, feelings, and thoughts

Look after others, offer them your listening ear and practical help where possible

Be part of a community and develop a sense of belonging, for example in the collective care process

Keep using your usual prescription medications

Recognise feelings of stress, anxiety, sadness, and notice that many people have similar experiences: these can be normal feelings in abnormal situations

Share your emotions with others, and create an (online) support network

Avoid being alone for long times

Do not discriminate or blame groups or individuals

Separate the place where you work from where you sleep (do not work or watch TV in bed) to prevent associating bed with being awake

Focus on activities that feel meaningful; plan at least one daily meaningful activity that you can look forward to

Take pride in small achievements, and in the fact that you have already been able to get through this difficult period so far

When talking with children: do not hide information, explain the situation in accessible language, keep a routine, maintain family routines, leisure time and games, be understandable of emotional changes and frustrations, limit the exposure to frightening news, stimulate physical exercise and sports

Be kind towards yourself: e.g. you do not need to do more than you are already doing (as some people are putting pressure on themselves by saying 'I must grow and learn something positive from the pandemic')

Prevent creating a large psychological threshold preventing you from going outdoors and meeting people, for example by regularly going into your garden or going to a nearby store; set safe and reasonable goals in small steps, reward yourself for small successes and be kind to yourself if you are not always successful

Double-check your thoughts: how realistic are your ideas? What do health authorities say?

Learn new skills, e.g. via online courses or YouTube videos or TED talks

Make a plan of what you could do if you were to become ill, and who could help you

Take time for creativity and expressing yourself, e.g. via making art, poems, writing, music

Reflect on what is really important in life and what your values are; how could you engage in meaningful and valuable activities in the present

Table 6.2 (Continued)

Recommendations

Reflect on your situation from the perspective of human history, in connection with others, in the past, present and future

Focus on how you can contribute to a just and ethical world

Find inspiration in mindfulness exercises, spirituality, or religion

Be grateful for small moments in life, albeit for the fact that you are alive

Make plans for the future, also beyond the pandemic

Table 6.3 Recommendations to health authorities for maintaining public mental health

Recommendations

In all communications about the pandemic, be honest about uncertainties and explain how the current strategy may be the best in the current situation

Care for the carers in words and actions: show health-care workers your respect, provide them with the resources and protective equipment they need

Create a culture of trust, openness, and transparency with health-care workers; ask for and value bottom-up input

Provide places where health-care workers can support each other, e.g. coffee rooms or online

Prepare, prepare, prepare: create contingency plans for a wide range of scenarios (small/medium/large crisis), buy required resources, and train all relevant health-care workers and civil servants

Show empathy and understanding for uncertainty, stress, anxiety, and outrage; be genuinely open for suggestions and make required changes

Emphasise the normality of feelings of uncertainty, stress, anxiety, and outrage

Create and spread psycho-educational material, particularly about how to cope with self-isolation and anxiety

Create multidisciplinary teams at the national level (e.g. SAGE), regions (e.g. cities, councils) and local health services

Facilitate a wide variety of volunteer work opportunities during lockdown, also online

Provide training in psychological self-care, debriefing, support networks and professional mental health-care for frontline workers

Provide training in identifying and assessing clients with mental health problems

Provide training in stress management, and protocols for working with trauma, anxiety, depression and risk behaviour

Provide large-scale screening for psychological problems for patients and their carers, e.g. at accident and emergency departments, intensive care units, general practitioner offices, care homes, and in other vulnerable populations

(Continued)

Table 6.3 (Continued)

Recommendations
Provide a diversity of mental health-care options, with a particular focus on trauma, grief, humanistic and existential care
Provide the facilities to supply mental health-care online, e.g. video, phone, apps, websites
Have one clear website from the health-care services, with clear information and guidelines
Encourage scientific research, not only biomedical but also behavioural and social research
Address inequalities in the physical and economic impact
Respect cultural differences, and provide culturally sensitive information
Prevent social isolation of vulnerable populations, e.g. individuals in care homes or psychiatric wards; create opportunities for (online) social contact, routine, and meaningful activities
Collect epidemiological data for research and future policies

7

EXISTENTIAL RISKS

UNCERTAIN LIFE

'The meaning of life is just to be alive. It is so plain and so obvious and so simple. And yet, everybody rushes around in a great panic as if it were necessary to achieve something beyond themselves. Life is not a problem to be solved, but an experience to be had.' (Watts,1951, p.25)

OVERVIEW

How much uncertainty can we bear? How much uncertainty can I bear – and how much can you? This seems to be a central question in this book as there are so many uncertainties. There are scientific uncertainties about the basic data of infection and mortality rates, and about the effects and unwanted side effects of herd immunity and quarantine. These uncertainties are embedded in a broader public debate about the status of research, due to its intertwining with commercial and political interests. There are uncertainties about the neutrality of governmental decision-making processes, with suspicions of corruption, and commercial use of the state of exception and the shock doctrine. Criticasters have raised fundamental doubts about the structural political causes of this pandemic, due to the ecological collapse and lack of preparedness, which seem to follow from a capitalist short-term-oriented political mindset. In this context of uncertainties and suspicions, several governments seemed to have played safe by imposing a strict lockdown, which may have slowed down the spread of the virus, but which may have also had significant adverse side effects – a tricky balance between two evils. Other governments have considered the option of herd immunity, but this option raised scientific and ethical doubts and was overhauled by the idea of nationwide lockdown. Communications from scientists and health authorities have created uncertainties, which seemed to be exacerbated by misinformation from the media and conspiracy theorists.

All these uncertainties, political failures and lack of preparedness seem to have led to the mental health impact of the pandemic on health-care workers, patients, and the general population. The body and the mind seem to have been working in tandem, with physical influences on people's emotional life, and high psychological stress levels influencing the functioning of the immune system and the subsequent susceptibility for infection by SARS-CoV-2. However, as we have seen, this psychological impact can only be understood from the context of interactions between the body, mind, and the socio-economic and political uncertainties. This mental health impact needs to be understood from the ways in which individuals have shaped their risk-perceptions and precautionary behaviours in response to these uncertainties. Individuals seem to have created their subjective interpretations of the pandemic, fuelled by media, friends, family, and culture.

Thus, if we want to go to the heart of the psychology of COVID-19, we need to explore how people experience and cope with uncertainty. In Chapter 1, we found a negative definition of 'uncertainty': uncertainties regarding the lack of conclusive answers and definitive solutions. Inherently, the science and politics of pandemics are full of uncertainties, as we are not speaking about the certainty that everyone in a population will get ill, but about the risks of infection and mortality. Whereas uncertainties are inherent to science and politics, non-specialists often seem to have the expectation – or the hope – that scientists and politicians could provide certainties. However, this may be like demanding the impossible. In this chapter, we will examine how people experience uncertainties in daily life, and how they wish for certainty – and how they cope when this wish remains unfulfilled. We will also examine the existential threat that uncertainties may bring, how people cope with this, and how people can live a meaningful and satisfying life despite the uncertainties.

PHENOMENOLOGICAL MODEL: UNCERTAINTIES IN DAILY LIFE

In everyday daily life, we rarely reflect on our body and our health risks. We simply follow our habits (Bourdieu, 1984). We are submerged in our subjectively lived experience of our body as part of the flow of our daily life (Vos, 2020, 2016, 2014). Only when our body stops working, or if we see an immediate

Table 7.1 Existential models, descriptions and COVID-19 examples

Existential model	Description	COVID-19 examples
Phenomenology	In our daily lives, we are often unaware of our bodies and our risks. When we become ill or our health risks are communicated to us, we may exchange this daily life gaze for a medical gaze towards ourselves. Unexpected life events, uncertainties, diseases, and health risks could make us reflect on our bodies, ourselves and our lives in general.	Some research studies and case reports suggest that individuals may experience their bodies in a different way and may reflect on their bodies, selves and lives. More research is needed.
Wish for certainty	Individuals can differ from each other in the extent to which they wish certainty in life, and in the extent to which they perceive the current situation as uncertain. The unfulfilled wish for certainty seems to explain the perception, behaviour, and mental health impact of health risk communication.	The more tolerant individuals are for uncertainties, the lower their levels of mental health problems are during the pandemic. However, more research is needed.
Existential threat	A pandemic can make individuals aware of existential themes in life, such as mortality, freedom, responsibility, social isolation and connectedness.	Research shows how individuals report reflections and moods related to the existential threat of COVID-19. However, more research is needed.
Terror management theory	The confrontation with disease and health risks may remind individuals of their mortality, which could trigger existential moods such as existential anxiety. Individuals could deny and avoid these reminders of their mortality – and thus improve their mood – via rationalisation or via shifting their attention to their worldview and meaning in life.	Individuals seem to cope with the existential threats of COVID-19 via rationalisation and attention-shifting. However, more research is needed.
Meaning-oriented coping	Individuals may have many ways to live a meaningful and satisfying life despite the uncertainties and existential threats of pandemics. The ability to live a meaningful life can help as a buffer to stress and a source of resilience.	Individuals who experience life as meaningful report more accurate risk perception, more flexible coping and better mental health. Social meanings and moral values are associated with a more frequent use of PPE, physical distancing and self-isolating.
Existential education	Individuals develop their perceptions, coping styles, and existential defence mechanisms in interaction with their upbringing, their social, political and economic context. Education may play an important role in learning to cope with risks, uncertainties and existential challenges.	More research is needed to understand the development and role of existential education during pandemics.

danger to our health, may we stop our habits and start reflecting or acting. In that situation, our relationship with our body may change: the habitual non-reflected flow of experiencing our daily life gets replaced by theoretical reflection or immediate action. We start looking at our body as an object that has nothing to do with us subjectively; we look with the eyes of an outsider at ourselves, like a doctor who looks with a medical gaze at a patient. The philosopher Martin Heidegger (1927) differentiated this medical gaze to our body – *Körper* in German – from our subjectively lived experience of the body – '*Leib*'. As Merleau-Ponty (1982) wrote: 'We understand the world from our phenomenological experience of our body.'

In contrast with this lived experience of our body, health risks are abstract, anonymous, and dehumanised (Castel, 1991): we reflect on the theoretical likelihood that our body – *Körper* – may become ill and how we might control these risks, for example by frequent hand-washing and self-isolation. The negative side is that, whereas our body was an unquestioned part of our lived experience before, we may now feel alienated from our body and treat it as a potential time bomb for ourself and others. The positive side is that this abstract way of self-reflection allows us to rationally control our behaviour and enables the authorities to survey our health and behaviour.

However, reflecting on our corporeal risks with a medical gaze seems to ignore the inherent meaning of the dangerousness of the pandemic for my *Leib*. That is, I reflect on the risks and I want to prevent these risks because I am afraid that I may lose my life, and I want to stay alive. My bodily experience (*Leib*) is entwined with my experience of life: my bodily experience is 'lived', and it is this lived experience of my body that is at stake during pandemics. Agamben (2017, p.56) writes that this lived experience of the body has only become a more common focus in politics and the population in general during the last few centuries; for example, the Ancient Greek word for the body also meant corpse, and thus the concept of life was absent from our way of speaking about the body. The medical gaze does not seem to do justice to the fact that my life may be at stake. Intriguingly, the modern word *Leib* is also etymologically derived from the German word for life, *Leben*: in our daily life, our bodily experience is part of our general experience of our life. 'This immediately brings mortality and finitude into our bodily experience: our body is about life and the absence of life – death. Our body is not merely a machine that can be eternally repaired and replaced; it is a limited being. Our internal experience of our finitude cannot be done justice in biomedical terms. We cannot objectively look, as a medical doctor does, at the expiry date of our body because we have our own subjective experience of it as an embodied being that is fragile and that will die one day. The biomedical approach lacks a perspective on this subjective experience of being limited in time, stretching between birth and death' (Vos, 2020, p.319).

This seems to explain why some people seem to panic when they are communicated infection risks: these are not merely neutral risks for them, but they feel that these risks mean direct danger to their life. 'Consequently, governments that impose a lockdown on their citizens also seem to impose existential anxiety. People become afraid of going outside, not merely because they do not want to break the rules but because they are afraid of getting or spreading COVID-19 and ultimately of suffering and death – even though they may not be aware of their existential motivations. This is what Heidegger (1927) calls *Angst*, being confronted with the fact that our body can fail and die, which can provoke a feeling of threat and anxiety. Stay home and save lives, that is what our governments tell us, and we do so because of the angst their message provokes' (Vos, 2020, p.319).

However, it is not certain that I will die now during this pandemic. I will certainly die one day, but I am still uncertain when and where that will be. This uncertainty about my death can be frightening. Some individuals may prefer the certainty of illness over the existential uncertainty. As we will see in the next section, people often feel scared to death by death. A good example is a 30-year-old woman who had an uncertain risk of developing breast and ovarian cancer due to uncertain heredity of cancer in her family (Vos, 2011). She asked her brother-in-law, who happened to be a surgeon, to preventatively remove her ovaries and breasts. This had a significant impact on her life, as she immediately came into the menopause and she could no longer have children, even though she did not have any children and her big dream in life had always been to become a mother. However, when she did a DNA-test afterwards, she found out that she did not have an increased risk of developing cancer after all. When I asked her how she felt about having her breasts and ovaries removed even though it was not medically necessary, she told me that she felt right about this: 'the certainty of having them removed is better than the uncertainty of keeping them; it was not certain that the DNA test would turn out this way.' The certainty of removing her 'time-bombs' – ovaries and breasts – was more important than the uncertainty of getting cancer, even though that would have allowed her to fulfil her life's dream. Similarly, people seem to think, feel, and act during the COVID-19 pandemic as if they are already ill, even though they have no symptoms and do not belong to a vulnerable population. Simultaneously, others seem to pretend that there are no risks at all, and do not use any PPE while ignoring the lockdown.

It seems as if people respond in black-or-white ways to the uncertainties of the pandemic, as if they find it difficult to tolerate these uncertainties. As we will see in the next section, people often respond in such black-or-white ways to existential uncertainties.

A pandemic can make individuals aware of themselves and of their fundamental approach to life. Will I try to look at the health risks with the medical gaze, pretending they are not about life and death? Will I listen to the authorities, or will I create my subjective interpretation independent from them? Am I OK with facing my vulnerability and mortality, or do I feel mortified and is that why I look away? Do I recognise that the risks are not only about my mortality but also the life and death of others – my risk-taking behaviour could put your life in danger in our highly interrelated world? What is my responsibility for others, what are my values? And if I recognise that the health risks limit my life, what shall I focus my limited time and energy on? Should I continue chasing meaningless projects like money and my career, or should I focus on what matters most to me, such as other people, connections, bigger life projects? Or are these existential questions too big – possibly because I feel unfulfilled about how I have lived my life so far – and therefore I pretend that my life is not at stake during this pandemic and I will deny the health risks? Any of these questions may arise as the pandemic can make us aware of our biomedical body, Life, Self and Being (Heidegger 1921/1995, GA21, pp.52–9). The next sections will review empirical studies supporting and rejecting this phenomenological approach to the risks and uncertainties during the COVID-19 pandemic.

'The worst of the self-isolation is the terror of boredom. My concept of time has changed – it feels long and dreary. The boredom feels so heavy because there is so much I want to do, and I do not know whether I will have enough time and opportunities in life to achieve everything I want. Will there be a post-COVID-19 future that will offer me these opportunities? The more bored I feel, the larger do I feel inner unrest, and do I want to explore the world outside. Recently, I had a nightmare: I was stuck in a boring life situation, and whatever I tried I could not escape the boredom – like in a Kafkaesque novel. The terror of boredom puts me in limbo: shall I break the self-isolation or shall I stay in?' (Interviewee Kevin)

UNFULFILLED WISH FOR CERTAINTY

The key to understanding the psychology of COVID-19 lies in understanding how individuals wish for certainty and how they perceive the uncertainties regarding COVID-19. Research has shown that individuals differ in their wish for certainty in different aspects of their lives (Vos, 2011). For example, some individuals seem to be wanting complete certainty about the infection risks, mortality risks, treatment options, and prevention, whereas others seem fine with some uncertainties. Some individuals see COVID-19 as a colossal disaster whereas others downplay all risks.

Often, there is a gap between the amount of certainty that individuals wish to have, and the certainty that they do have: an unfulfilled wish for certainty. It is the fulfilment of this wish for certainty that seems to explain how individuals perceive and respond to COVID-19. For example, the more unfulfilled someone's wish for certainty is, the more black-or-white it is: *I want certainty, and therefore I assume that nothing serious is going on and the full pandemic is just a hoax,* or: *I want certainty and therefore I assume that this pandemic will be the end of humanity.* The more someone's wish for certainty remains unfulfilled, the more stressed, anxious, and depressed they will be (Vos, 2020, 2011): *I desperately want to know what is going on, but I do not, and therefore I am stressed!* This is what research on COVID-19 showed: the better individuals can tolerate uncertainty, the better is their mental health (Larsen et al., 2020; Satici et al., 2020; Rettie & Daniels, 2020; Tull et al., 2020; Vazqueza et al., 2020). Thus, individuals differ in how they cope with the lack of fulfilment of their wish for certainty. For example, the more uncertainties individuals have experienced previously in their lives, the less stressed they feel about uncertainties in the present, and the less black-or-white is their perception. The more meaningful life feels to individuals, the less stress and the less black-or-white perception will they experience regarding COVID-19. These findings make sense: when someone has learned how to live a meaningful and satisfying life despite life's uncertainties, the more resilient will their reaction be when facing new uncertainties such as COVID-19.

EXISTENTIAL THREAT

Our wishes and perceptions of uncertainties regarding different domains in life differ from each other (Vos, 2011). For example, I might want a lot of certainty over the likelihood that I might get infected by COVID-19 but I can perceive that I do not have much certainty over this; the stress that I may experience over this lack of uncertainty may be different than, for example, the uncertainty that I have about the future popularity of this book. I can live better with not knowing whether this book will be a success than with not knowing whether I will get infected with COVID-19, and ultimately with not knowing whether

COVID-19 will kill me or not. As we have seen in the phenomenological analysis above, our lived experience of our body immediately brings in an existential perspective; the uncertainty about my health and mortality matter more to me than, for example, the uncertainty about my book's success, because this is about Me, my Life, my Being. It is this existential nature of uncertainty that seems to make COVID-19 so stressful.

In the literature review, I found 13 studies on the existential meaning of COVID-19. These studies indicate that COVID-19 can be an immediate threat to the ability to sustain oneself due to financial uncertainty and unemployment (Blustein & Guarino, 2020) and to one's social context (Ufearoh, 2020). Individuals may start to realise that the world is not as explainable, controlled and benevolent as they had once thought (De Jong et al., 2020; Trzebiński et al., 2020). Individuals can also feel confronted with the limits of life with topics such as life/death and freedom/responsibility (Bland, 2020). In other words: pandemics can be stressful because they confront us with our general human condition. That is, the pandemic could shatter the fundamental illusions that they have in daily life and make individuals aware of universal facts about life. For example, individuals could feel that they are thrown onto themselves: although they may receive support from friends, colleagues, and relatives, they realise that they have to get through health risks and sickness themselves, and nobody else could take over *their* health risks for them. Ultimately, individuals are responsible for their perception and response to the health risks and their health or illness, and this could give rise to a sense of existential loneliness.

More specifically, COVID-19 can undermine individuals to engage in behaviour that they had deemed meaningful before, such as sports, going out or any other activities that are hindered by self-isolation. COVID-19 can also cast individuals out of their habits and make them reflect on what is truly meaningful in life. Individuals who are aware of what makes their life meaningful, also report lower levels of psychological stress during COVID-19, possibly because the sense of meaningfulness makes them more resilient and flexible to adjust to existential challenges; these individuals may even experience a sense of growth during the pandemic (Arslan & Yildirim, 2020; Bojanowska et al., 2020; Lau et al., 2020; Nowicki et al., 2020; Yang, 2020; Yu et al. 2020). I also found in my survey the double conclusion that most individuals experience the pandemic as an existential turning-point, and those who experience life as meaningful seem more flexible in coping with the pandemic and report lower levels of psychological stress (Vos, 2020b).

TERROR MANAGEMENT THEORY: COPING WITH EXISTENTIAL THREAT

We have seen how COVID-19-related uncertainties can feel as existential threats. How do people cope with this existential threat? To answer this question, we will explore the Terror Management Theory (TMT), which has been developed by Sheldon Solomon, Jeff Greenberg and Tom Pyszczynski (2015), in response to the book *Denial of Death* by Ernest Becker (1974). TMT has been supported by thousands of empirical studies in many different populations, including people facing existential health risks. Several studies on COVID-19 have also confirmed this model (e.g. Bottemanne et al., 2020; Courtney et al., 2020; Menzies & Menzies, 2020).

The basis of TMT is simple. Like all animals, human beings want to live – Agamben sees naked *Biological Life* as a starting point (2020). Therefore, anything that makes them think about the end of life makes them anxious. This is existential anxiety – angst – which is not about a specific object – like a phobia is, for example, about snakes or spiders – but this is about the fear of losing life as such. We have two ways of setting this existential anxiety aside, and both ways may be the result of our upbringing and socialisation (Greenberg et al., 2014).

First, we can use so-called proximal defence mechanisms, which are about any rational or superficial ways of stopping reminders about death. For example, individuals may rationalise the infection risks of COVID-19 by arguing that they do not have an underlying physical vulnerability. Thus, people may change their perception of COVID-19 so that it does not feel existentially threatening anymore. COVID-19 may be a threat to someone else, but not to me. Research on the denial of health risks shows that these types of denial and avoidance of risks may work in the short term; however, in the long term, avoidance and denial seem to break down as they become more and more unrealistic (Vos, 2011).

Second, we can use so-called distal defences – possibly after the proximal defences have failed. These defence mechanisms work by shifting the attention to one's worldview and meanings in life. One example is that individuals may start to defend their worldview, even at the cost of others. In response to the existential threat of COVID-19, individuals have become more conservative (Rosenfeld & Tomiyama, 2020), xenophobic (Bartos et al., 2020; Emanuel et al., 2020) and sinophobic (Tabri et al., 2020). People explore fewer varieties, for example, in the supermarket, when they feel existentially threatened during COVID-19 (Kim, 2020). To trigger these proximal or distal defence mechanisms, the existential threats by COVID-19 do not need to be realistic such as the risk of unemployment and financial upheaval, but can be purely imagined and, for example, regard one's socio-cultural identity (Kachanoff et al., 2020). TMT is relevant for health authorities, as individuals may respond to the existential anxiety triggered by COVID-19 by performing less preventative behaviours. For example, Jimenez et al. (2020) found that individuals who associated COVID-19 with death were less likely to use PPE or go into physical isolation; they suggested that too much existential threat in the communications from health authorities may therefore be counterproductive.

MEANING IN LIFE

Thus we see that the COVID-19-related uncertainties could feel like an existential threat, which individuals could push away through cognitive strategies or shifting their attention to their worldview. Racism, xenophobia, and hoarding may all be regarded as examples of TMT.

A concept related to worldviews is 'meaning in life'. People often speak about the importance of meaning when they are confronted with life's boundaries, such as the threat of chronic or life-threatening disease (Vos, 2016). The concept of meaning-oriented coping has become widely used in the field of health psychology, as many studies have shown how individuals can try to negotiate the meaning of a health risk with their meaning in life. That is, they could find new ways to live a meaningful and satisfying life despite the limitations that the health risks pose to them. For example, the family could be an important source of meaning for someone, but the lockdown has made it difficult to meet up in person; although it is not the same as meeting IRL, meeting online with their relatives could still give a sense of meaning.

It is easy to get stuck in the role of being a patient or being a person at risk. Individuals may fall into a vicious cycle of the patient role: they simply lie in bed, become obsessed with any news and information about COVID-19, become hyper-anxious, hyper-vigilant and hyper-observant about any physical unease, which makes them feel worse and motivates them even more to avoid any social and physical activities. However, each individual has a meaningful potential that reaches beyond the patient role: we are children, parents, employees, partners, friends, music-lovers, etc. The patient role has taken over all other roles. Patients have described how they need to remind themselves of these other forgotten roles actively. 'You need to have some normal things. You cannot lie in bed all day every day. Albeit a big physical struggle, I force myself to do things that feel meaningful, such as going to the local park, even if that is only for 20 minutes' (COVID-19 patient Mary).

These moments may help clients to go beyond the vicious cycle of being a patient and being nothing else than a patient. Experiences that go beyond the present and offer a larger perspective ('transcendence'). Research shows that explicitly focusing on meaningful roles and activities during physical illness ('meaning-oriented coping') can lead to better mental and physical health, including improved functioning of the immune system, less pain, and faster physical recovery (Vos, 2016).

The psychotherapist Alfried Langle concluded in this context: 'Meaning is always possible, also during COVID-19' (IMEC Conference, 25 July 2020, meaning.org.uk). With this formulation, he rephrased the words of the father of the field of logotherapy ('logo' = meaning) and existential analysis. Viktor Frankl had been imprisoned in the concentration camp at Auschwitz, and he had observed how individuals who were able to experience any meaning in life were the ones who would survive. Giving up the belief that meaning is possible means giving up life. Therefore, Frankl originally entitled his best-selling book about his camp experiences 'Saying Yes to Life Despite Everything', which was later changed into *Man's Search for Meaning*. He discovered that humans could cope with the biggest tragedies in life, as long as they focus on what is meaningful to them. Of course, the way we fulfil our meaning may look different when we are limited. For example, Frankl could not meet his wife in person, but his image of her in his mind kept him going. This core idea – focusing on meaning can help to cope with existential threats – has been proven in countless studies. For example, the dominant theories in health psychology seem to recognise the importance of meaning, albeit with different terms: individuals struggle with chronic or life-threatening physical diseases due to the challenges to their sense of meaning, and their ability to experience meaning despite these challenges makes them more mentally resilient and helps them to cope (Vos, 2016). Similarly, during the COVID-19 pandemic, we may not be able to realise our meanings in life in the same way as we did before, but we can try to realise our most important meanings in life in new ways.

What is meaning in life? Meaning should not necessarily be understood in theoretical or philosophical terms such as 'The Meaning of Life', like with a philosophical gaze. The meaning that I am referring to is about the lived experience of Life as being meaningful (Vos, 2020, 2018, 2016). It is not a noun but an adjective, as it describes our way of living meaningfully. Research indicates that meaning in life is about having goals, directions or motivations, values, commitment, understanding of your context, feeling worthy of following your own meanings, and the ability to set goals and navigate flexibly through life when confronted with existential challenges. This can be realised in many different ways. Research shows that across the globe, individuals usu-ally experience six types of meaning: materialistic, hedonistic, self-oriented, social, larger, and existential-philosophical types of meaning. Usually, indi-viduals have a combination of meanings, and the more meanings one has, the more flexible one is to cope with adversity; for example, if a person has work as the sole meaning in life and they are put on furlough or made redun-dant, they may then feel that life is meaningless and not worth living. Social and larger types of meaning are also associated with better mental health, whereas materialistic, hedonistic, and self-oriented types are associated with relatively lower mental health.

Therefore, it did not come as a surprise that in my survey, individuals who had three or more types of meaning, and who dominantly focused on social and larger types of meaning, seemed more resilient in coping with COVID-19: they experienced less psychological stress, although they recognised the sever-ity and existential nature of COVID-19. The more individuals experienced life as meaningful, the better were they able to accept the COVID-19-related uncer-tainties, and the more were their interpretations in line with the government's recommendations (Vos, 2020). This is in line with previous studies showing that individuals who experienced life as meaningful had more accurate risk-perceptions, showed more flexible coping-styles and experienced better men-tal health in confrontation with health threats (Vos, 2011). Having a sense of meaning in life seems to work as a buffer against existential anxieties, frustra-tions and outrage that may arise in response to existential uncertainties and threats such as COVID-19. Studies across the globe have confirmed that the presence of meaning in life is associated with more accurate risk-perception, more flexible coping and better mental health during the COVID-19 pandemic (Arslan & Yildirim, 2020; Bojanowska et al., 2020; De Jong et al., 2020; Lau et al., 2020; Nowicki et al., 2020; Trzebiński et al., 2020; Tyner & Rice, 2020; Yang, 2020; Yu & Li, 2020; Yu et al., 2020).

EXISTENTIAL EDUCATION

TMT suggests that individuals may learn their existential defence mechanisms from their parents and society. As babies and children, we are vulnerable and depend on the protection from adults, and thus we will try to obey to our caregivers in the hope that they will protect us, even though they may not always actually do that, as in the case of emotional neglect or sexual abuse. Whatever our situation is, we are likely to be trying to appease our caregivers, and to do so we try to show behaviour and express values that they praise and reinforce. Consequently, we internalise the worldviews of our caregivers, without necessarily asking for the justifications or truth behind this worldview. Our worldviews are our defence mechanisms against existential terror, the fear that we could be factually, symbolically, or imaginarily left alone by our protectors. Thus, it seems that we start protecting what we have never consciously and deliberately considered meaningful. We will be loyal to those who have given us the light of life and who had protected us when we were the most vulnerable, whatever happens (Boszormenyi-Nagy, 2013).

In our upbringing, we often seem to learn that uncertainty equates to danger. In the worst case, it is the danger of our direct and indirect protectors – from our parents to our governments – turning against us. The mere thought of lacking their approval and support can trigger rigid defence mechanisms, pushing away any uncertainties, ambiguities, or ambivalences. Even though in Reality – and beyond our hopes and expectations – our protectors are individuals who are as vulnerable as we are and who have internalised their parents' worldviews. Therefore, it may not be surprising that – in line with our existential certainties – our education system was communicating in terms of certainties and truths; at school, we rarely learn things that The Grown-Ups do not know or about which they feel uncertain. Teachers seem to rarely show human Reality by telling us that they do not know something, or that they feel uncertain or insecure. Thus, we develop the expectation that life is full of certainties, and we develop the habit that, when confronted with uncertainties, we either dismiss the uncertainties or we turn towards our protectors – our literal or symbolic parents – to internalise how they transform the uncertainties into certainties. Without realistic and critical education, children may grow up as adults with unrealistic expectations about themselves, life and the world around them (Vos et al., 2019).

HOW TO CREATE EXISTENTIAL RESILIENCE

This chapter has summarised how uncertainty seems to be at the heart of the COVID-19 crisis that society is facing. Often, we do not want these uncertainties, as we want to be certain at least about the fundaments of our life, such as our ability to stay physically healthy, feed ourselves and have a roof over our heads. However, the pandemic pulls these assumptions into uncertainty, as we may become ill, we may lose our job, and we may lose our house. Thus, although we may not be aware of it in our daily life, the COVID-19 uncertainties can refer back to the existential possibility that we can die now from the pandemic and the existential certainty that we will die one day in future. As we do not like to be confronted with our mortality – as we strive to stay alive – we may try to minimise the risks that COVID-19 poses to us cognitively, and we may submerge ourselves in our worldview and become conservative or defensive of our values and meaning in life. However, when we focus on authentic meaning – not meaning as a defence mechanism, but in line with what feels like our 'true self' (Schlegel et al., 2009) – we may also be able to tolerate the uncertainties and the existential threats. That is, authentic meaning can help us to face uncertainties and existential boundary situations, without feeling so overwhelmed that we activate our proximal or distal existential defence mechanisms.

On a phenomenological level, uncertainties seem to be about emptiness: the loss of meanings or opportunities, and a confrontation with the ultimate emptiness of life – death (Vos, 2018, 2014). Therefore, it is not surprising that several clients and participants describe how COVID-19 has made their lives feel empty. The question is: are we able to transform this sense of emptiness into a sense of space? Can we change the emptiness from old meanings into space for new meanings? As Heidegger (1927) wrote: being-alive – being-there – is being-in-possibilities (*Dasein ist Dasein-konnen*); we have time and space to change. How will we play around in our time-play-space? How will we use our opportunities? Will we use the opportunities to be authentic or inauthentic?

The existential author Albert Camus shows these existential mechanisms very clearly in his book *The Plague* (1948). Although the book is fiction, the examples he gives seem very close to our existential responses to COVID-19. In this book, some individuals respond authentically to a pandemic of the plague: they acknowledge their uncertainties and limitations, do not pretend to be better or worse than they are, and they try to follow their ethical values. Others, however, choose an inauthentic response, deny the existential threats, and use the uncertainties to their advantage, for example by focusing on marketing and selling their products in times of shortage. This is the fundamental decision that each of us has to make: will we respond in an authentic or inauthentic way to the pandemic?

8

THE WORLD RESILIENCE SOCIETY

'The desire for security and the fear of insecurity are the same thing. To hold your breath is to lose your breath. A society based on the quest for security is nothing but a breath-retention contest in which everyone is as taut as a drum and as purple as a beet.' (Watts, 1951)

FROM WORLD RISK SOCIETY TO WORLD RESILIENCE SOCIETY

We live in a World Risk Society: we are continuously reminded of risks around us, from the financial risks of our loans and mortgages to climate change. Out of all the possible risks that could have brought society to a standstill, it was the SARS-CoV-2 virus with a mere size of 0.00012 millimetres that did. Similar to many other societal risks, the risks that this virus brings us are surrounded with uncertainties, from the questions that people have asked about the basic data collection to the governmental recommendations about face-masks, herd immunity and quarantine.

Similar to other risks, people seem to hate the uncertainties related to the COVID-19 pandemic. However, in this context of uncertainties, some health authorities seem to have decided to transform the reality of uncertainties into imaginary or symbolic certainties, at least in their communications. Unknowns are presented as knowns. This transformation is not extraordinary as, in general, people seem to have the psychological tendency to respond in black-or-white ways to uncertainties, as we have seen in previous chapters. Some people even seem to prefer the certainty of suffering or death over having to live with uncertainties. Individuals may tell themselves and others satisfying stories full of certainties about the pandemic, even though they may be aware that the scientific and political reality beyond these imaginations and symbolic stories is much more uncertain. The existence of so many uncertainties combined with the human wish for certainties seem to have created opportunities for both well-intending scientists and bad-intending crooks. Like the pharmaceutical company which used the 1918 pandemic to sell carbolic smoke balls, companies seem to be selling their hopes for COVID-19 tests, treatments and vaccines, even though these have not always been fully developed or tested for their side effects, while governments, for example, need to take over the liability for adverse side effects. Thus, there may be nothing unique about the COVID-19 risks, its existential uncertainties, and our human dislike of these uncertainties. Possibly the difference is the large scale of the denial of uncertainty during a pandemic, and its consequences for the economy and individual physical and psychological health.

The solution for our pandemic crisis of uncertainty may be the creation of new ways to live a meaningful and satisfying life while being realistic about the certainties and uncertainties, and the building of meaningful communities to support each other in coping with our shared and personal certainties and uncertainties. Only this attitude of being realistic about our certainties and uncertainties may help us to transform what sociologists call our 'World Risk Society' into what I call a 'World Resilience Society'. Elsewhere, I have named this World Resilience Society a Meaning-Oriented Society (Vos, 2020), and both terms seem exchangeable, as a sense of meaning in life can give us an intuitive compass, leading us away from meaningless uncertainties into the direction of meaningful opportunities, as we have seen in a previous chapter.

In the next sections, I will ask ten different questions about how the World Risk Society and the World Resilience Society address or could address pandemics. These ten questions follow from the Systematic Pragmatic Phenomenological Approach, which is a systematic and critical way to develop an in-depth understanding of a social phenomenon (Vos, 2020, 2020d). In these analyses, I will go beyond the direct observations and systematic research, to give an initial sketch of some broader trends, although some trends will need further elaboration and research. This chapter will finish with questions for health authorities and individuals. The core questions will be: how much uncertainty can you bear? Which meaningless uncertainties could you transform into meaningful opportunities?

THE WORLD RISK SOCIETY

Epidemiologists and virologists predict that there will be more pandemics in future, mainly as a consequence of ecological collapse and global hyper-connectedness (Chapter 4). This also implies that there may be more 'Second

Pandemics' of political, socio-economic and psychological responses to the bio-medical pandemics. Consequently, our world may not be as safe, controllable, and understandable as we may have assumed in the past, and there may be an end to our myth of unlimited economic progress. Instead, we may learn how the world also bears risks, uncertainties, and possible socio-economic decline.

Already more than a decade before COVID-19, the sociologist Ulrich Beck has described our era as the 'World Risk Society', and Zygmunt Bauman called it a 'Liquid Society'. They fundamentally characterised our era as dominated by risks and uncertainties, such as health risks, economic risks, and the risk of climate change. However, the concept of the World Risk Society seems to have been hijacked by Third Way sociologists and politicians such as Anthony Giddens, Tony Blair and Bill Clinton, who have made risks into something controllable and manageable via pseudo-neoliberal methods, such as outsourcing research, privatising risks, and privatising national services (Vos, 2020). For instance, their administrations removed researchers from governmental departments, and seemed to ignore research reports calling to prepare for pandemics. Thus, their approach seemed to show the danger of denying risks or shifting of risk management to private players such as pharmaceutical companies who sell a story of perfect control.

Status of our knowledge: We have seen in Chapter 2 that the science of COVID-19 is extraordinary science, with an unclear intertwining of science, governments, global health organisations, and commercial interests. This seems to have led to questions about a lack of preparedness, uncertain data, and uncertainties about the two main strategy options of herd immunity and quarantine. Thus, scientific reality seems to be filled with uncertainties. Of course, when I write 'reality' here, this is a relative term; as fallible human beings with our limited senses and instruments, we may never be able to understand the Ultimate Reality – if there is something like that; we can only have our best guesses about reality. If scientists or government press officers aimed to do justice to Ultimate Reality, they would also have been communicating how many uncertainties there are, and how much we do not know. However, anyone watching the daily briefings from the press rooms in the White House or 10 Downing Street may have only been observing a Platonic shadow show – mere tragi-comedic entertainment or Hollywood drama? – devoid of the reality of uncertainties, human errors, and individual differences? Although this may be an extreme depiction of these press briefings, it seems that the denial of uncertainties has forced press officers into a tango of bending and twisting, giving explanations for the unexplainable, and broadcasting certainty where there is none. The Emperor is naked, but we do not seem to be saying this aloud.

The psychoanalyst Jacques Lacan made a difference between Reality and reality, and he suggested that the latter (reality) is our symbolic and imagined construction of how Reality may look. Symbolisation and imaginations of Reality are nothing extraordinary, as they are part of our daily interactions and communications. However, problems seem to occur when influential individuals structurally communicate that their symbols and imaginations are the sole Reality, that people need to follow their Commandments, and that anyone violating the Law is a risk and thus needs to be quarantined – just like anthropologists wrote about hygiene practices, and how the Thora book of Exodus spoke about the exclusion of 'the unclean'. Although many governmental recommendations during the pandemic seem sensible given the scientific status quo, the ontological conflation underlying the governmental communication seems to exclude the realistic possibility of doubts and lack of clarity. The more uncertain politicians are, the more they seem to communicate in terms of certainty, ranging from populism and fascism to Corona Capitalism (Vos, 2020). Understandably in response to this conflation, citizens may start to not only doubt the message but also the messenger: they seem to criticise governments and scientists and develop their own Conspiracy Theories. Therefore in several countries, the pandemic seems to have led to an ontological crisis in political legitimacy.

Materialistic and self-oriented types of meaning: We have seen how scientists and governments often seem to look with a biomedical gaze to the pandemic, whereas the subjectively lived experiences of our body and its associated risks transcends this gaze in our everyday daily life. Thus, it seems as if this pandemic reduces the dynamic and complex totality of our subjectively lived experiences of our own body into a single materialistic object, casting out any individual variations and subjectively lived experiences. *But I am more than a potential time bomb of SARS-CoV-2; do not treat me as a soulless object! No, you are not! Wear a face-mask and obey the social distancing rules, or we will lock you up!* Although all government communication may always have some reductionist tendencies – as states need to use generalised communication and may not be able to do justice to each individual citizen – this dehumanised materialistic gaze seems in line with the materialistic focus of neoliberalism and modern neoliberal communism like in China (Vos, 2020).

Neoliberalism is not merely an approach to economics, but also a framework to what citizens may see as meaningful in life. We saw for instance how the British minister Keith Joseph wrote how politicians may need to actively push the general population to accept the materialistic and self-oriented focus of neoliberalism (Vos, 2020). Joseph suggested that any collective experiences may be used for manipulation of the mindset of citizens, ensuring that they will support neoliberal values. Some criticasters have hypothesised that in a similar spirit, some of the government approaches to COVID-19 seem to impose a reductionist gaze on materialistic and self-oriented meanings, offering a shock doctrine for preachers of materialism and self-care. We may hypothesise that it is unsurprising that commercial companies frame the pandemic in mere materialistic terms, potentially stimulating a self-oriented competitive spirit of all against each other. The term 'herd immunity' may also be indicative of this dehumanisation and stripping the individual of their subjectively lived experiences, as the individual – the *Homo Sacer* – may need to be sacrificed for the herd. The argument for nationwide lockdowns seems similarly focused on the biomedical risks and seems to ignore the significant psychological and social side effects of self-isolation, and thus cast the complex totality of individuals into potential viral vessels and time bombs.

Functionalistic approach: We have seen how materialism seems to go hand in hand with a functionalist approach: COVID-19 is a material thing – albeit of microscopic size – that can and *should* be controlled (is/ought-fallacy?). Individual citizens become part of dehumanised functions – such as the epidemiological SIR-model – which do not do full justice to the social and larger meanings that COVID-19 may have to individuals. There is no such thing as certainty for model-makers: any statistical model inherently involves risks and uncertainties. However, the overall likelihood and variance accounted for by the statistical models may disappear in their dehumanised translation and communication by politicians: *We know how to control this pandemic! We must take these precautionary measures, otherwise we are doomed!* Individual citizens are reduced to functions in the statistical functions of the state, and statistical variation and errors may be dismissed as necessary side effects.

Relationship between individual and society: The chapter on politics brought us to biopolitics, which are the ways governments govern biological phenomena and the biomedical dimension of citizen life. Biopolitics involves many variations and risks – as, by definition, a population does not have one physical body, but many individual bodies. The question is how governments manage the uncertainties associated with these. We saw how governments have responded to the COVID-19 pandemic by increasing their external control and authoritarian measures such as fining anyone who is not self-isolating or who is not wearing a face-mask in public spaces. We also saw how internal control (self-governmentality) was stimulated by appealing to the personal sense of responsibility, guilt, and shame of citizens.

Development over time: Why do individuals obey their governments? Hannah Arendt asked this question in her book *Eichmann in Jerusalem*, with the protagonist, Eichmann, who was responsible for coordinating the trains to concentration camps. Eichmann's life story struck Arendt as an ordinary father and responsible citizen, who thought that he was just following orders, and he claimed that he did not know precisely what happened in the camps. Thus, Arendt concluded that evil could be very banal, existing in tiny decisions in daily life situations, which – if taken on their own – do not seem evil at all. Arendt explained how a line of tiny steps might constitute Evil.

No reasonable moral comparison can be made between an individual coordinating trains to the Final Solution during the Second World War, and individual citizens believing and obeying the demands and recommendations of their health authorities during a pandemic. However, Arendt used Eichmann's case to describe the general societal mechanism of explicitly and implicitly indoctrinating individual citizens, while individuals may let themselves be indoctrinated by not being critical enough. We have, for example, seen how risk-perceptions, mental health and behaviour can be shaped over time by influences from government, scientists, the media, and the pharmaceutical industry. However, we have also seen how individuals can develop their interpretation, independently from whatever governments or media tell them. It seems to be in the small mundane steps of everyday life that individuals may develop their perception and response to the COVID-19 pandemic, and the underlying question seems to be how critical they are of those influencing them, and of their perceptions and behaviours. However, at the same time, what is the ability of citizens to separate the wheat from the chaff, governmental manipulation from wise advice; for example, how can individuals know whether it is wise to use PPE and go into self-isolation? Ultimately, the question is how practically and morally self-reflexive individual citizens are in their daily life during pandemics. However, we may not have the precise answer to these questions, as we are just facing hypotheses and uncertainties as individual citizens who may be unable to know what is precisely going on beyond the screens of biopolitics.

Who has power over whom: Chapter 3 outlined the inequality of the impact of COVID-19, as is often the case with epidemics. It seems that the pandemic – or even more broadly speaking, the World Risk Society – brings an inequality to the risks that different individuals in society carry, as the most vulnerable seem to bear the largest risks and the most uncertainties. It seems to be the inequality of power relationships that have led to large-scale demonstrations and social disruptions at the end of the pandemic in the most unequal Western countries, the USA and UK, as if COVID-19 were the final straw for these demonstrators.

What they seem to be demanding are democracy and equality – or better said: equity of opportunities in society. In contrast, the reconstruction of the societal response to the pandemics in this book has focused on the role of a relatively small group of influencers, mainly key governmental advisors, individual scientists, and pharmaceutical industries, which seems to leave out the voices of the many. Their perceptions and decisions have determined nationwide lockdowns and governmental communication, which has determined the citizens' risk-perception, psychological stress, mental health, and behaviours.

Sense of freedom: The philosopher Esposito has argued that governments have excluded individuals from society during the pandemic. For example, we have seen how 'risky' frontline workers or former patients feel stigmatised. We have also seen how the pandemic has in general led governments to limit the freedom of movement, the freedom of gathering in larger groups, etc. Thus, the uncertainty of risks seems to have brought some experiences of negative freedom, inequality, and powerlessness. In contrast, there has been little or no communication about positive freedoms, such as ways of helping each other during COVID-19, and how to live a meaningful and satisfying life despite the pandemic. This lack may be endemic of neoliberalism, which seems to focus on negative freedom – telling us what *not* to do – instead of positive freedom – facilitating people to do what they genuinely want to do (Vos, 2020).

Existential ground: 'Thou must change, or thou shalt die – or thy neighbour shall!' We could possibly say that rarely have modern societies seen such a large-scale existential campaign by governments. The World Risk Society is infused with existential messages, angst and existential defence mechanisms. Although we may want to think that we are unique, the current pandemic is not unique regarding our collective existential response, for example in the aftermath of the 9/11 attacks, the 7/7 London bombings, or the 2007/8 financial crash. We have always been at risk: these collective traumas have reminded us of our fragility, and in response, we become nationalistic, conformist or populist, and focus on what we think is the most valuable. Although these responses seem understandable, they do not seem to do full justice to the underlying feelings of existential vulnerability, mortality, and loneliness. Similarly, the COVID-19 pandemic seems to have triggered feelings of conservatism, populism, or even outright fascism, almost forgetting the underlying foundations of risks and uncertainties.

Impact on daily life: Living in the World Risk Society seems to be associated with risks and uncertainties that we did not want to know, and while casting these risks and uncertainties away from our consciousness, we seem to be creating mental health problems, low quality of life and poor life satisfaction.

Our mental health seems to be in a collective crisis, and our mental health authorities may not be able to give an efficient response as they may be stuck in their socio-economic-political position (Vos et al., 2019). Consequently, the standard mental health-care solutions that health services offer may only scratch the surface and help clients to create their own certainties, while leaving out the realistic topics of risks and uncertainties (ibid.).

THE WORLD RESILIENCE SOCIETY

Whereas the above-mentioned sociologists such as Ulrich Beck seemed to dominantly focus on the negative sides of risks, we could also explore how we could develop a 'World Resilience Society'. This is a society in which individuals do not see risks only as problems but also as opportunities – both at the same time: a dual attitude (Vos, 2020, 2018, 2014) – and where individuals can live a meaningful and satisfying life despite acknowledging the realistic risks, transforming existential emptiness into space (Vos, 2014). In the following paragraphs, I will fall into a logical is/ought-fallacy from how things are to how things should possibly be: we may restructure economics and politics – and we are already seeing such trends – in such a way that we embrace uncertainties and become more resilient against future shocks while giving a clear black-or-white response after any systematic evidence-based research. This pandemic could give us the opportunity and hope for a Big Reset of our socio-economic and political system (Schwab & Malleret, 2020).

Status of our knowledge: Whereas the World Risk Society seems to have focused on symbolic and imaginary risks to go around Real risks and uncertainties, the World Resilience Society acknowledges – and may even embrace – risks and uncertainties. This means that, throughout their decisions and communications, scientists and governments mention the risks, variations and uncertainties involved; their communication is transparent and facilitates critical public debate. If they present any symbols or imaginings – which is inevitable as we humans seem to desire these – they are explicit about their ontological status: this is our vision, not Reality. Education should include modules to help children, young people, vulnerable individuals – and possibly the general population – to develop critical thinking skills, to differentiate Reality from symbols and imagination.

Types of meaning: Although its starting point is the plurality of perspectives and meanings in society, the World Resilience Society predominantly focuses on social and larger types of meanings (Vos, 2020). This means that social and ethical values, the sense of community and altruism, may predominate any decisions from governments and health authorities. We do not merely need to limit the biomedical risks of COVID-19, but also the risks of social division, a me-versus-the-rest mentality, mass unemployment and devaluation of employee skills. If we want to control the First – biomedical – Pandemic, we also need to cope with this Second Pandemic of individual and social psychological processes. Ultimately, the question is: what type of society do we want to be? Do we want to be exclusive for healthy able individuals who fit our right psychological and socio-economic framework, or do we want to be inclusive?

General approach: Whereas functionalism – reducing individuals to anonymous variables in a statistical function – is inherent to mathematical-biomedical and neoliberal approaches to COVID-19, a critical-intuitive – or phenomenological – approach determines the World Resilience Society. This approach takes the inherent meaningfulness of individuals as a starting point. This means that government policies should not only do justice to the largest number of individuals as possible but go beyond this, as no groups will be structurally excluded. Variations and uncertainties are acknowledged and explicitly communicated – they are not regarded as a threat or variation to the mean but as opportunities and synergies. This also implies specific strategies and communications to specific communities, particularly those at high risk, such as individuals with a low socio-economic status or black and minority ethnic (BAME) background: the one size of governmental policies does not fit all. Several populist – or semi-fascist – political leaders seem to have rejected national diversity; however, their policies seem divisive and contra-productive, especially when public health is at risk: an epidemic in one specific community can quickly jump onto another community. Inclusive politics may reduce the risks that a local or regional outbreak spirals down into a pandemic. This may require both vertical and horizontal aid strategies from international health organisations such as the WHO.

Relationship between individual and society: Whereas we have seen that a relatively small elite of governmental decision-makers and scientists seem to make the critical decisions and communications regarding public health in the World Risk Society, the World Resilience Society is characterised by a more bottom-up, proactively empowering approach to democracy. This implies the creation of mutual trust between authorities and the public. This is a two-sided process, as the public seems to mistrust authorities, and authorities seem to mistrust the general public in neoliberal countries. Scandinavian countries are an example of relative mutual trust between authorities and public, where authorities trust the common sense of people, for example regarding self-isolating when there are significant signs or risks, such as any symptoms of COVID-19 or having an underlying vulnerability or being in touch with vulnerable individuals.

The core question is: who carries the principal risks and uncertainties, and what is the role of the state in the context of a less hierarchical, citizen-led approach to governance? How can we share responsibilities with realistic accountability procedures as part of the public dialogue, and not merely in legal terms? How can we learn to build relationships and communities? How can we build mutual trust between citizens in their governments and leaders and vice versa? Which type of dialogue could create this trust? This may require bold new answers. For example, research suggests that countries with female leaders who are quicker in deciding about nationwide lockdowns and who have shown more empathy in their communications and strategies have been more successful in reducing their COVID-19 infection and mortality risks than countries with male leaders who have one-sidedly imposed their COVID-19 measures (Aldrich & Lotito, 2020; Sergent & Stajkovic, 2020). Thus, we may need a bottom-up democratic approach to pandemics, with open interaction between individual citizens and authorities, where a critical attitude is stimulated, and a diversity of voices is heard.

Development over time: Many chapters have described how our perceptions, mental health and behaviours can be shaped by a range of individuals who seem to have their interests primarily at heart. A World Resilience Society offers the teaching of education of critical thinking skills. These skills may help us understand and critically interpret risk communication by authorities, companies, and lobbyists. Whereas the UK – with other Western countries following in its footsteps – seem to have focused their education on market-relevant skills – as the neoliberal minister Keith Joseph argued that teaching critical thinking skills will not give neoliberal parties a majority – the World Resilience Society offers education that includes critical thinking and existential skills (Vos et al., 2019). Critical pedagogy would include psycho-education about our human wish for certainty, and how sometimes in life we cannot achieve certainty and that we should not fall for false prophets promising certainties in these uncertain periods. On a political level, corruption and nepotism should be fought, including a ban on lobbying by pharmaceutical companies who seem to have significantly influenced prior governmental and intergovernmental decisions regarding pandemics. We have also seen the dangers of science becoming dependent on commercial funding; therefore, non-commercial funding should guarantee the independence of research.

Who has the power over whom: We have seen how in our current World Risk Society, undemocratic processes may have influenced individual perceptions, mental health and behaviours. In contrast, the World Resilience Society facilitates building bottom-up proactive democracy, mutual trust, empowerment of individuals, the expression of a diversity of voices, and the creation of sharing communities. These are very generic formulations, and it may be easy to give the nod to these sentences; however, the practice of creating a bottom-up participatory democracy can be hard but rewarding work in practice.

Sense of freedom: Isaiah Berlin (1959) differentiated negative freedom from positive freedom. Negative freedom implies that we are not allowed to do certain things – like being in public without a face-mask – whereas positive freedom implies an active stimulation of individual opportunities. The latter includes examples such as ways in which we can stay socially connected during lockdown, how we can democratically contribute to decision-making about the pandemic, what could we do to support each other during this pandemic. We have seen relatively few examples of governmental communication about positive alternatives to how individuals could live a meaningful and satisfying life despite the pandemic.

Existential ground: This book has shown how a lack of existential realism may have determined our collective and individual responses to COVID-19. We often seem to be wanting certainty, while in Reality we are confronted with many uncertainties. As research suggests, there are three ways to cope with this. Either we lower our wish for certainty regarding COVID-19, we lower the uncertainties we perceive (for example, reinterpret the situation by focusing on certain aspects), or we try to find certainty in our generic meanings in life (such as shifting our attention from the existential threats to our worldviews, relationships and activities that we experience as meaningful). The concentration camp survivor and psychiatrist Viktor Frankl called this attitude tragic optimism: while recognising the tragedy that is happening in Reality, remaining optimistic about the opportunity of better times, and actively searching for – and actively creating opportunities of – meaningful moments in life. This is a 'dual awareness', which is the simultaneous awareness of our existential Reality as well as our opportunities for meaning, however small these meanings may be in everyday life (Vos, 2014). For media and governments, this implies that not only the existential dangers of the pandemic should be communicated, but also positive opportunities for people to live a meaningful life and support each other in meaningful communities.

Impact on daily life: Whereas the World Risk Society seems to be associated with mental health problems, a low quality of life and life-satisfaction, a World Resilience Society may possibly offer mental well-being, good quality of life and life-satisfaction. This is because meaning-oriented coping skills are stimulated, which are known to be effective in stimulating a realistic assessment of the situation as well as reasonable behaviour and good mental health (see previous chapter). However, it seems to be a figment of the imagination that life could ever be totally problem-free; all of us will confront inevitable challenges in life, even in a low-risk Walhalla (Vos et al., 2019). Therefore, it will be essential to help people develop realistic expectations about life and to provide psycho-education about how to cope with life's challenges and uncertainties.

'A new politics of uncertainty must challenge the biopolitical framings and governmentalities of conventional technocratic approaches that define populations or geographic areas as "at risk". Instead, the intersections of uncertainty, vulnerability, precarity and marginalisation must be taken seriously, alongside a commitment to "cognitive justice". This suggests a very different type of approach, centred on shared understandings, the negotiation of outcomes and collective solidarity and mobilisation. It must be rooted in what we have earlier identified as a politics of care and conviviality, rejecting a simple reliance on state protection, standardised welfare and market-based insurance. Asking questions about whose crisis, catastrophe or emergency it is, and how it is experienced, is not a denial of the importance of the event, or the roles for expertise in defining key aspects. Instead, it is a recognition that climate change, disease, earthquakes – or other uncertain events – will look different from the standpoint of those living in conditions of precarity and vulnerability. This means recasting responses, moving away from those that are forged through externally-imposed, expert-led governmentality towards forms of "response-ability", with located capabilities and horizontal accountabilities at the core.(...)

Such explorations of everyday uncertainties and how people negotiate them amid precarious lives start to open up different, and richer, understandings of uncertainty as it relates to disease outbreaks. These understandings involve moves from context to text; from epistemology to ontology; from individual/ community perspectives to social relational ones; and from narrow temporalities (the immediate outbreak, the future plan) to multiple ones, as past, present and imagined future dynamics inform each other. Perhaps above all, they suggest that uncertainties are not always amenable to being reduced to risk, and managed and controlled – and that, furthermore, attempts at control may simply spawn further uncertainties. The reality of a multitude of forms of uncertainty, temporalities and experiences does not mean that we should dismiss the urgency of outbreak response, or suggest that efforts to research pathogens, engage with models and predict and indeed prepare for epidemics are not important. Understanding everyday uncertainties and their implications for epidemic preparedness and response must emerge from continuous engagement, as responses to such lived uncertainties can be revealing of local efforts that are of relevance for outbreak preparedness.' (Scoones & Stirling, 2020, pp.17–18,121–2)

POLITICAL ACTIVISM

The big question is: how could the World Risk Society transform into a World Resilience Society? There are clear indications that this transformation is currently happening (e.g. Schwab & Malleret, 2020; Vos, 2020). For example, over previous decades, citizens seem to have become more critical of governments and make their decisions based on what they deem to be inherently meaningful. In this regard, COVID-19 seems to have a Janus-face: on the one hand, some individuals seem to have been following the communications from governments and scientists uncritically, but on the other hand – particularly during lockdown – some individuals have started to reflect on what matters in their own lives and society in general. For example, several countries have seen demonstrations against the supposed authoritarianism and unequal structural policies of their governments, including the Black Lives Matter movement. In the UK and the USA, critical masses of parents have refused to send their children to school after the lockdown, as parents seem to question both the safety and the quality of the education.

A sense of existential urgency is often the crucial spark for an uprising in the population (Engler & Engler, 2018). When individuals feel threatened in their existence, they will be willing to put more at risk to demonstrate and demand justice for their case – or similar cases. As explained in previous chapters, COVID-19 may offer the ultimate existential spark for uprisings. Although some uprisings have been recorded – particularly in the USA – the lack of large-scale uprisings in other countries seems telling – which may be due to a pacifying Corona Life Syndrome.

Let us examine what research tells about existential activism. Research indicates that individuals are more likely to support and participate in social movements when there is a combination of factors (Vos, 2020): deprivation of social and larger types of meaning; if a political campaign has social and larger meanings as campaign aims and methods; if counter-propaganda is well-framed; and if there are sufficient practical resources for the movement. A good example is the uprising of the Black Lives Matter movement at two-thirds of the pandemic, which was initially triggered by the killing of the Black man George Floyd by police officers, and which at a later stage pulled in many others dissatisfied about inequalities in society regarding wealth and health. For example, COVID-19 has revealed structural existential injustices, for example regarding health-care providers, physically vulnerable individuals, socio-economic inequalities, unsupportive education systems. Political campaigns are most likely to be effective when they address a wide range of meanings, particularly social and larger meanings, when they are not too functionalist, underline existential urgency, psychologically empower activists, and connect the meanings of the campaign with the meanings of powerholders (Vos, 2020).

Furthermore, research suggests that if social movements are to be effective, they may need to focus on the deprivation of social and larger types of meaning, have social and larger meanings as campaign aims, use social and larger meanings as campaign methods, have meaningful propaganda and framing – and be prepared to counter the fake news from the counter-revolution movements – and have sufficient resources. The movement needs to have a positive identity, stating clear political aims and ideological position about each of the ten meaning-oriented perspectives (Vos, 2020). The future will tell us whether and which movements will effectively arise out of the COVID-19 pandemic.

HEALTH AUTHORITIES

This book has provided many suggestions for health authorities, such as governmental decision-makers, advisors, and health-care coordinators. Chapter 6 has provided a table with specific recommendations. However, what has not been addressed is a change in attitude. We could approach the pandemic with the perspectives of either the World Risk Society or the World Resilience Society; which approach do governments want to take? Research suggests that the more capitalist, male-dominated and less-empathic governments are – at least in their communications – the higher are their infection and mortality rates for COVID-19 (Aldrich & Lotito, 2020; Martinez, 2020; Sergent & Stajkovic, 2020; Vos, 2020a). Thus, the question is not only about how governments could communicate effectively about COVID-19, but how they should structurally change themselves in such a way that they do not merely contribute to the creation of the pandemic – e.g. via ecological collapse and global traffic – but that they help the creation of a resilient society.

INDIVIDUALS

We have encountered many differences between individuals in how they experience and respond to COVID-19. There is not a one-size-fits-all approach to the most effective way to cope as an individual with COVID-19. Chapter 6 has provided a table with suggestions, but these seem to only scratch the surface. The main question is: how much uncertainty do you dare to bear, and how do you want to respond to our complex Reality of certainties *and* uncertainties? What will you do to make a difference, for yourself and others? These are the questions that will determine our future. The choice is yours.

Table 8.1 Characteristics of World Risk Society and World Resilience Society

Question	Description	World Risk Society	World Resilience Society
Status?	Status of our knowledge	Symbolic and imagined control over symbolic and imagined certainties (need for certainty)	Complex, dynamic reality with management of certainties and uncertainties (acceptance of certainties/uncertainties)
What?	Types of meaning	Materialistic and self-oriented types of meaning	Holistic, focus on social and larger types of meaning
How?	General approach	Functionalistic	Critical-intuitive
Where?	Relationship between individual and society	External control (authoritarianism) and internal control (self-governmentality); biopolitics	Critical-empathic societal dialogue, acknowledging of risks and uncertainties
When?	Development over time	Risk-perceptions, mental health and behaviour are shaped over time by influences from government, scientists, the media and the pharmaceutical industry, while critical thinking is destimulated	Psycho-education and critical interpretation skills education from young age onwards, fight corruption and nepotism, stimulate independent science
Who?	Who has the power over whom	A small elite of governmental decision-makers and scientists make decisions which influence citizens' risk-perception, psychological stress, mental health, and behaviour	Bottom-up proactive democracy, build trust, empowerment, resilience-building, critical-thinking, diversity of voices, sharing communities
Whose?	Sense of freedom	Negative freedom, inequality, helplessness	Positive freedom, equality, empowerment
Why?	Existential ground	Existential angst and existential defence mechanisms	Existential realism
Which?	Impact on daily life	Mental health problems, low quality of life, low life satisfaction	Mental well-being, good quality of life and life satisfaction

REFERENCES

Abate, B. B., Kassie, A. M., Kassaw, M. W., Aragie, T. G. & Masresha, S. A. (2020). Sex difference in coronavirus disease (COVID-19): A systematic review and meta-analysis. *BMJ Open, 10*(10), e040129.

Abeysinghe, S. & White, K. (2010). Framing disease: The avian influenza pandemic in Australia. *Health Sociology Review, 19*(3), 369–81.

Agamben, G. (2017). *The Omnibus Homo Sacer.* Redwood, CA: Stanford Press.

Agamben, G. (2020a). The invention of an epidemic. *European Journal of Psychoanalysis.* May. www.journal-psychoanalysis.eu

Agamben, G. (2020b). The state of exception provoked by an unmotivated emergency. *Positions Politics.* May. www.positionspolitics.org

Aggarwal, N., Dwarakanathan, V., Gautam, N. & Ray, A. (2020). Facemasks for prevention of viral respiratory infections in community settings: A systematic review and meta-analysis. *Indian Journal of Public Health, 64*(6), 192–9.

Ahmad, A. R. & Murad, H. R. (2020). The impact of social media on panic during the COVID-19 pandemic. *Journal of Medical Internet Research, 22* (5), e19556. doi:10.2196/19556

Aldana, S. G., Sutton, L. D., Jacobson, B. H. & Quirk, M. G. (1996). Relationships between leisure time physical activity and perceived stress. *Perceptual and Motor Skills, 82*(1), 315–21.

Aldrich, A. S. & Lotito, N. J. (2020). Pandemic performance: Women leaders in the Covid-19 crisis. *Politics and Gender,* 1–9.

Allcott, H., Boxell, L., Conway, J., Gentzkow, M., Thaler, M. & Yang, D. Y. (2020). *Polarization and Public Health,* NBER Working Paper, w26946. doi: 10.3386/w26946

Allington, D., Duffy, B., Wessely, S., Dhavan, N. & Rubin, J. (2020). Health-protective behaviour, social media usage and conspiracy belief during the COVID-19 public health emergency. *Psychological Medicine,* 1–7.

Andersen, K. G., Rambaut, A., Lipkin, W. I., Holmes, E. C. & Garry, R. F. (2020). The proximal origin of SARS-CoV-2. *Nature Medicine, 26* (4): 450–52.

Anderson, B. (2010). Preemption, precaution, preparedness. *Progress in Human Geography, 34* (6): 777–98.

Aradau, C. & Van Munster, R. (2011). *Politics of Catastrophe.* Abingdon: Routledge.

Arafat, S. Y., Kar, S. K., Marthoenis, M., Sharma, P., Apu, E. H. & Kabir, R. (2020). Psychological underpinning of panic buying during pandemic. *Psychiatry Research, 289*: 113061–70.

Arendt, H. (1973). *The Origins of Totalitarianism*. Boston, MA: Houghton Mifflin Harcourt.

Armstrong, G. (2020). The Billionaires Behind the Crisis. Eyes on the Ties. News. littlesis.org

Arndt, J., Solomon, S., Kasser, T. & Sheldon, K. M. (2004). The urge to splurge. *Journal of Consumer Psychology, 14* (3): 198–212.

Arslan, G. & Yildirim, M. (2020). Meaningful Living, Resilience, Affective Balance, and Psychological Health Problems during COVID-19. Preprint: https://psyarxiv. com/wsr3e/

Atchison, C. J., Bowman, L., Vrinten, C., Redd, R., Pristera, P., Eaton, J. W. & Ward, H. (2020). Perceptions and behavioural responses of the general public during the COVID-19 pandemic: A cross-sectional survey of UK Adults. *medRxiv.*

Atkinson, D. & Elliott, L. (2008). *The Gods that Failed: How Blind Faith in Markets Has Cost Us Our Future*. London: Random House.

Baddeley, M. (2020). Hoarding in the age of COVID-19. *Journal of Behavioral Economics for Policy, 4* (S): 69–75.

Banerjee, D. (2020). The other side of COVID-19: Impact on obsessive compulsive disorder (OCD) and hoarding. *Psychiatry Research, 288*: 112966–71.

Barrios, J. M. & Hochberg, Y. (2020). Risk-perception Through the Lens of Politics in the Time of the Covid-19 Pandemic (w27008). National Bureau of Economic Research.

Barry, J. M. (2009). Pandemics: Avoiding the mistakes of 1918. *Nature, 459* (7245): 324–5.

Bartos, V., Bauer, M., Cahlíková, J. & Chytilová, J. (2020). *Covid-19 Crisis Fuels Hostility Against Foreigners*. Preprint: https://papers.ssrn.com/

Bauman, A. E. (2004). Updating the evidence that physical activity is good for health: An epidemiological review 2000–2003. *Journal of Science and Medicine in Sport, 7*(1), 6–19.

Bauman, Z. (1990). Modernity and ambivalence. *Theory, Culture and Society, 7* (2–3): 143–69.

Bechtel, B. R. & Berning A. (1990). *The Third-quarter Phenomenon*. New York: Springer.

Beck, U. (2009). World risk society and manufactured uncertainties. *IRIS 1* (2): 291–310.

Beck, U., Giddens, A. & Lash, S. (1994). *Reflexivity Modernization*. Redwood, CA: Stanford Press.

Becker, E. (1974). *The Denial of Death*. New York: Simon and Schuster.

Benson, V. S., Pirie, K., Schüz, J., Reeves, G. K., Beral, V. & Green, J. (2013). Mobile phone use and risk of brain neoplasms. *International Journal of Epidemiology, 42* (3): 792–802.

Berger, J. & Milkman, K. L. (2012). What makes online content viral? *Journal of Marketing Research, 49* (2): 192–205.

Berkman, L. F., Kawachi, I. & Glymour, M. M. (2014). *Social Epidemiology*. Oxford: Oxford University Press.

Berlin, I. (1959). Two concepts of liberty: An inaugural lecture delivered before the University of Oxford on 31 October 1958 (Vol. 31). Oxford: Clarendon.

Berry, J. M. & Sobieraj, S. (2013). *The Outrage Industry: Political Opinion Media and the New Incivility*. Oxford: Oxford University Press.

Betrus, M. (2020). *Lockdowns on Trial*. Independently published.

Best, P., Manktelow, R. & Taylor, B. (2014). Online communication, social media and adolescent wellbeing: A systematic narrative review. *Children and Youth Services Review, 41,* 27–36.

Bibby, J., Everest, G. & Abbs, I. (2020). *Will COVID-19 Be a Watershed Moment for Health Inequalities*, The Health Foundation. May. www.health.org.uk

Biddlestone, M., Green, R. & Douglas, K. (2020). Cultural orientation: Powerlessness, belief in conspiracy theories, and intentions to reduce the spread of COVID-19. *British Journal of Social Psychology, 59* (3): 663–73.

Biondi, M. & Zannino, L. (1997). Psychological stress, neuroimmunomodulation, and susceptibility to infectious diseases in animals and man: A review. *Psychotherapy & Psychosomatics, 66*(1), 23.

Bird, S. E. (1996). CJ's revenge: Media, folklore, and the cultural construction of AIDS. *Critical Studies in Media Communication, 13* (1): 44–58.

Bish, A. & Michie, S. (2010). Demographic and attitudinal determinants of protective behaviours during a pandemic. *British Journal of Health Psychology, 15* (4): 797–824.

Bish, A., Yardley, L., Nicoll, A. & Michie, S. (2011). Factors associated with uptake of vaccination against pandemic influenza: A systematic review. *Vaccine, 29* (38): 6472–84.

Bishop, M. & Green, M. (2010). *Philanthrocapitalism*. New York: Bloomsbury.

Bjørkdahl, K. & Carlsen, B. (eds) (2018). *Pandemics, Publics, and Politics: Staging Responses to Public Health Crises*. Gateway East, Singapore: Springer. doi: 10.1007/978-981-13-2802-2

Bjørkdahl, K. & Carlsen, B. (2019). *Pandemics, Publics, and Politics*. Singapore: Palgrave Pivot.

Bland, A. M. (2020). Existential Givens in the COVID-19 Crisis. *Journal of Humanistic Psychology, 60*(5), 710–24.

Blustein, D. L. & Guarino, P. A. (2020). Work and unemployment in the time of COVID-19: The existential experience of loss and fear. *Journal of Humanistic Psychology, 60*(5), 702–9.

Bodenheimer, T. (2000). Uneasy alliance: Clinical investigators and the pharmaceutical industry. *New England Journal of Medicine, 1539*: 1540–54.

Bojanowska, A., Kaczmarek, Ł. D., Kościelniak, M. & Urbańska, B. (2020). *Values and Well-being Change Amidst the COVID-19 Pandemic in Poland*. Preprint: https://psyarxiv.com/xr87s/

Boland, H. & Zolfagharifard, E. (2020). Coding that led to lockdown was totally unreliable and a buggy mess. *The Telegraph*, 16 May.

Boroush, M. (2015). U.S. R&D increased in 2013. *National Science Foundation InfoBrief*. 22 July.

Boszormenyi-Nagy, I. K. (2013). *Between Give and Take*. London: Routledge.

Bottemanne, H., Morlaàs, O., Schmidt, L. & Fossati, P. (2020). Coronavirus: Predictive brain and terror management. *L'encephale, 46* (3S): S107–S113.

Bourdieu, P. (1984). *Distinction*. London: Harvard University Press.

Bourgeois, F. T., Murthy, S. & Mandl, K. D. (2010). Outcome reporting among drug trials registered in K. Bowman, K. & A. Rugg (2013). Five years after the crash: What Americans think about Wall Street, banks, business, and free enterprise. *American Enterprise Institute Public Opinion Studies.* Available at www.aei.org/wp-content/uploads/2013/09/-five-years-after-the-crash-what-americans-think-about-wall-street-banks-business-and-free-enterprise_083339502447.pdf (Accessed on 15 October 2020).

Bowman, K. & Rugg, A. (2013). Public opinion on conspiracy theories. *AEI Paper & Studies.*

Brady, J., Iwamoto, D. K., Grivel, M., Kaya, A., & Clinton, L. (2016). A systematic review of the salient role of feminine norms on substance use among women. *Addictive Behaviors, 62,* 83–90.

Brewer, N. T., Chapman, G. B., Gibbons, F. X., Gerrard, M., McCaul, K. D. & Weinstein, N. D. (2007). Meta-analysis of the relationship between risk-perception and health behavior. *Health Psychology, 26* (2): 136.

Brooks, S. K., Webster, R. K., Smith, L. E., Woodland, L., Wessely, S., Greenberg, N., & Rubin, G. J. (2020). The psychological impact of quarantine and how to reduce it: Rapid review of the evidence. *The Lancet.* [Epub ahead of print]

Brown, R. M. (2009). *Animal Magnetism.* New York: Ballantine.

Brown, T. I., Gagnon, S. A. & Wagner, A. D. (2020). Stress disrupts human hippocampal-prefrontal function during prospective spatial navigation and hinders flexible behavior. *Current Biology, 30* (10): 1821–33.

Budrys, G. (2003). *Unequal Health: How Inequality Contributes to Health or Illness.* Lanham, MD: Rowman & Littlefield Publishers.

Burnside, R., Miller, D. S. & Rivera, J. D. (2007). The impact of information and risk-perception on the hurricane evacuation decision-making of greater New Orleans residents. *Sociological Spectrum, 27* (6): 727–40.

Business Insider (2020). How 'Professor Lockdown' helped save tens of thousands of lives worldwide – and carried COVID-19 into Downing Street. *Business Insider,* 25 April. www.businessinsider.com

Calman, K. & Curtis, S. (2010). *Risk Communication and Public Health.* Oxford: Oxford University Press.

Campbell, K. K. & Jamieson, K. H. (2006). The interplay of influence: News, advertising, politics, and the internet. *Public Relations Review, 32* (1): 88–9.

Camus, A. (1956/2012). *The Plague.* London: Vintage.

Cargile, J. (1997). On the burden of proof. *Philosophy, 72* (279): 59–83.

Carr, P. R. (2020). If everything has changed, why such a focus on bailing out capitalism? *Postdigital Science and Education, 1*: 1–7.

Carrington, D. (2020). UK strategy to address pandemic threat not properly implemented. *The Guardian,* 29 March.

Case, A. & Deaton, A. (2020). *Deaths of Despair and the Future of Capitalism.* Princeton, NJ: Princeton University Press.

Cassam, Q. (2019). *Conspiracy Theories.* Hoboken, NJ: John Wiley & Sons.

Cassam, Q. (2020). *The Metaphysical Foundations of Vice Epistemology.* London: Routledge.

Castel, R. (1991). From dangerousness to risk. In G. Burchell, C. Gordon, & P. Miller (eds) (1991). *The Foucault Effect: Studies in Governmentality*: 281–9.

Cheng, S. K. W., Tsang, J. S. K., Ku, K. H., Wong, C. W. & Ng, Y. K. (2004). Psychiatric complications in patients with SARS during the acute treatment phase. *British Journal of Psychiatry*, *184* (4): 359–60.

Chetty, T., Daniels, B. B., Ngandu, N. K. & Goga, A. (2020). A rapid review of the effectiveness of screening practices at airports, land borders and ports to reduce the transmission of respiratory infectious diseases such as COVID-19. *South African Medical Journal*. [Epub ahead of print]

Chlan, L. & Savik, K. (2011). Patterns of anxiety in critically ill patients receiving mechanical ventilatory support. *Nursing Research*, *60*(3 Suppl), S50.

Chu, D. K., Akl, E. A., Duda, S., Solo, K., Yaacoub, S., Schünemann, H. J., ... & Hajizadeh, A. (2020). Physical distancing, face masks, and eye protection to prevent person-to-person transmission of SARS-CoV-2 and COVID-19: A systematic review and meta-analysis. *The Lancet*. [Epub ahead of print]

Clark, D. A. (2004). *Cognitive-Behavioral Therapy for OCD*. New York: Guilford Press.

ClinicalTrials.gov. *Annals of Internal Medicine*, *153* (3): 158–66.

Clinton, C. & Sridhar, D. (2017). *Governing Global Health: Who Runs the World and Why?* Oxford: Oxford University Press.

Cochrane. (2011). How well do meta-analyses disclose conflicts of interests in underlying research studies. *Cochrane*. www.cochranelibrary.com

Cohen, S. (1996). Psychological stress, immunity, and upper respiratory infections. *Current Directions in Psychological Science*, *5* (3): 86–9.

Cohen, A. N., Kessel, B. & Milgroom, M. G. (2020). Diagnosing COVID-19 infection: The danger of over-reliance on positive test results. *medRxiv*.

Cohen, S., Tyrrell, D. A. & Smith, A. P. (1991). Psychological stress and susceptibility to the common cold. *New England Journal of Medicine*, *325* (9): 606–12.

Collinson, S., Khan, K. & Heffernan, J. M. (2015). The effects of media reports on disease spread and important public health measurements. *PloS one*, *10*(11), e0141423.

Coombs, W. T. (2014). *Ongoing Crisis Communication: Planning, Managing, and Responding*. London: Sage. Sage: London.

Corrard, F., Copin, C., Wollner, A. . . . & Cohen, R. (2017). Sickness behavior in feverish children is independent of the severity of fever. *Plos one*, *12* (3): e0171670.

Cosgrove, L., Karter, J. M., Morrill, Z. & McGinley, M. (2020). Psychology and surveillance capitalism: The risk of pushing mental health apps during the COVID-19 pandemic. *Journal of Humanistic Psychology*, *60*(5): 611–25.

Courtney, E. P., Goldenberg, J. L. & Boyd, P. (2020). The contagion of mortality. *British Journal of Social Psychology*, *59* (3): 607–17.

Cruwys, T., Stevens, M. & Greenaway, K. H. (2020). A social identity perspective on COVID-19: Health risk is affected by shared group membership. *British Journal of Social Psychology*, *59* (3): 584–93.

Dalmeet, S. C. (2020). Critiqued coronavirus simulation gets thumbs up. *Nature*, *582*: 323–4.

Dantzer, R., O'Connor, J. C., Freund, G. G., Johnson, R. W. & Kelley, K. W. (2008). From inflammation to sickness and depression. *Nature Reviews Neuroscience*, *9* (1): 46–56.

Dantzer, R. (2009). Cytokine, sickness behavior, and depression. *Immunology and Allergy Clinics*, *29*(2), 247–64.

Davey, M., Kirchgaessner, S. & Boseley, S. (2020). Surgisphere: Governments and WHO changed Covid-19 policy based on suspect data from tiny US company. *The Guardian*, 3.

Davidoff, F., Deangelis, C. D., Drazen, J. M. & Wilkes, M. S. (2001). Sponsorship, authorship and accountability. *CMAJ*, *165* (6): 786–8.

Davydow, D. S., Desai, S. V., Needham, D. M. & Bienvenu, O. J. (2008). Psychiatric morbidity in survivors of the acute respiratory distress syndrome: A systematic review. *Psychosomatic Medicine*, *70*(4): 512–19.

Davydow, D. S., Hough, C. L., Langa, K. M. & Iwashyna, T. J. (2013). Symptoms of depression in survivors of severe sepsis: A prospective cohort study of older Americans. *The American Journal of Geriatric Psychiatry*, *21*(9): 887–97.

De Genova, N. (2020). Life versus capital. *Social Anthropology*, *28* (2): 253–4.

De Jong, E. M., Ziegler, N. & Schippers, M. (2020). *From Shattered Goals to Meaning in Life: Life Crafting in Times of the COVID-19 Pandemic*, Preprint: repub.eur.nl

Dean, M. (2010). Power at the heart of the present. *European Journal of Cultural Studies*, *13* (4): 459–75.

Dean, M. (2014). Rethinking neoliberalism. *Journal of Sociology*, *50* (2): 150–63.

Deaton, A. (2013). *The Great Escape: Health, Wealth, and the Origins of Inequality*. Princeton, NJ: Princeton University Press.

Deleuze, G. (1995). *Control and Becoming and Postscript on Control Societies*. New York: Columbia University Press.

Della Rosa, A. & Goldstein, A. (2020). What does COVID-19 distract us from? *Social Anthropology*, *28* (2): 257–9.

Desclaux, A., Diop, M. & Doyon, S. (2017). Fear and Containment. In M. Hofman & S. Au (eds), *The Politics of Fear*. Oxford: Oxford University Press.

Devakumar, D., Shannon, G., Bhopal, S. S. & Abubakar, I. (2020). Racism and discrimination in COVID-19 responses. *The Lancet*, *395* (10231): 1194.

DHSC, ONS, GAD & HO. (2020). *Direct and Indirect Impacts of COVID-19 on Excess Deaths and Morbidity*. Department of Health and Social Care, Office for National Statistics, Government Actuary's Department and Home Office. 15 July.

Dobson, S. (2020). *Epidemic Modelling*. Independent Publishing Network.

Dohle, S., Wingen, T. & Schreiber, M. (2020). *Acceptance and Adoption of Protective Measures During the Covid-19 Pandemic*. Preprint: osf.io

Doshi, P. (2020). Will COVID-19 vaccines save lives? Current trials aren't designed to tell us. *British Medical Journal*, *371*: 4037.

Douglas, M. (1966/2013). *Risk and Blame*. London: Routledge.

Douglas, M. (1986/2003). *Purity and Danger*. London: Routledge.

Dryhurst, S., Schneider, C. R., Kerr, J. . . . & Linden, S. (2020). Risk-perceptions of COVID-19 around the world. *Journal of Risk Research*, *1*: 1–13.

Dyer, O. (2020). Covid-19: Black people and other minorities are hardest hit in US. *British Medical Journal*, *14* (369): 1483.

El-Gingihy, Y. (2018). *How to Dismantle the NHS in 10 Easy Steps*. London: John Hunt.

Elliott, R. (1997). Existential consumption and irrational desire. *European Journal of Marketing*, *31* (3/4), 285–96.

Emami, A., Javanmardi, F., Pirbonyeh, N. & Akbari, A. (2020). Prevalence of underlying diseases in hospitalized patients with COVID-19: A systematic review and meta-analysis. *Archives of Academic Emergency Medicine*, *8* (1): 1–25.

Emanuel, L., Solomon, S., Fitchett, G., Chochinov, H., Handzo, G., Schoppee, T. & Wilkie, D. (2020). Fostering existential maturity to manage terror in a pandemic. *Journal of Palliative Medicine*. Epub.

Engler, M. & Engler, P. (2016). *This is an Uprising: How Nonviolent Revolt is Shaping the Twenty-First Century*. New York: Nation Books.

Esposito, R. (2011). Immunitas: The protection and negation of life. *Polity*.

Evangeli, M., Pady, K. & Wroe, A. L. (2016). Which psychological factors are related to HIV testing? *AIDS and Behavior*, 20 (4): 880–918.

Farmer, P. (2003). Pathologies of power: Health, human rights, and the new war on the poor. *North American Dialogue*, 6 (1): 1–4.

Faulkner, J., O'Brien, W., McGrane, B. . . . & Elliot, C. (2020). *Physical Activity, Mental Health and Well-being of Adults During Early COVID-19 Containment Strategies*. Preprint: medRxiv.org

Ferguson, N., Laydon, D., Nedjati, G. . . . Ghani, A. (2020). *Impact of Non-pharmaceutical Interventions to Reduce COVID-19 Mortality and Health-care Demand. Report*. 16 March.

Fischhoff, B. (2003). Judged terror risk. *Journal of Risk and Uncertainty*, 26 (1): 137.

Fischhoff, B. (2012). Evolving judgments of terror risks. *Journal of Experimental Psychology*, 18 (1): 1.

Fitzgerald, M. & Crider, C. (2020). Under pressure, UK government releases NHS COVID data deals with big tech. *OpenDemocracy*: June 5.

Fletcher, R., Kalogeropoulos, A. & Nielsen, R. K. (2020). Trust in UK Government and News Media COVID-19 Information Down, Concerns Over Misinformation from Government and Politicians Up. *Reuters Institute*. 1 June.

Folkman, S. (Ed.). (2011). *The Oxford Handbook of Stress, Health, and Coping*. New York: Oxford University Press.

Folkman, S. & Lazarus, R. S. (1984). *Stress, Appraisal, and Coping* (pp. 150–153). New York: Springer Publishing Company.

Foucault, M., Agamben, G., Nancy, J. L. . . . & Carolis, M. (2020). Coronavirus and philosophers. *European Journal of Psychoanalysis*. March. https://www.journal-psychoanalysis.eu/coronavirus-and-philosophers/

Freestone, P. P., Sandrini, S. M., Haigh, R. D. & Lyte, M. (2008). Microbial endo-crinology: How stress influences susceptibility to infection. *Trends in Microbiology*, 16 (2): 55–64.

French, M. & Monahan, T. (2020). Disease surveillance. *Surveillance and Society*, 18 (1): 1–11.

Fries, J. F. & Krishnan, E. (2004). Equipoise, design bias, and randomized controlled trials: The elusive ethics of new drug development. *Arthritis Research and Therapy*, 6 (3): 1–6.

Fuchs, C. (2020). Everyday life and everyday communication in coronavirus capital-ism. *Communication, Capitalism and Critique*, 18 (1): 375–99.

Gao, J., Zheng, P., Jia, L. . . . & Dai, J. (2020). Mental health problems and social media exposure during COVID-19 outbreak. *Plos one*, 15 (4): e0231924.

Garbe, L., Rau, R. & Toppe, T. (2020). Influence of perceived threat of Covid-19 and HEXACO personality traits on toilet paper stockpiling. *Plos one*, 15 (6): e0234232.

Garfin, D. R., Thompson, R. R. & Holman, E. A. (2018). Acute stress and subsequent health outcomes. *Journal of Psychosomatic Research, 112*: 107–13.

Garikipati, S. & Kambhampati, U. (2020). *Leading the Fight Against the Pandemic: Does Gender 'Really' Matter?* Preprint: www.ssrn.com

Georgiou, N., Delfabbro, P. & Balzan, R. (2020). COVID-19-related conspiracy beliefs and their relationship with perceived stress and pre-existing conspiracy beliefs. *Personality and Individual Differences, 166*: 110201.

Glaser, R. & Kiecolt-Glaser, J. K. (2005). Stress-induced immune dysfunction: Implications for health. *Nature Reviews Immunology, 5* (3): 243–51.

Glik, D. C. (2007). Risk communication for public health emergencies. *Annual Review of Public Health, 28*: 33–54.

Godlee, F. (1994). The World Health Organisation: WHO in crisis. *BMJ, 309* (6966): 1424–8.

Goldacre, B. (2013). *Bad Pharma: How Drug Companies Mislead Doctors and Harm Patients.* London: Macmillan.

Goodwin, R., Wiwattanapantuwong, J., Tuicomepee, A., Suttiwan, P. & Watakakosol, R. (2020). Anxiety and public responses to COVID-19. *Journal of Psychiatric Research, 129*: 118–21.

Gøtzsche, P. (2013). *Deadly Medicines and Organised Crime. How Big Pharma Has Corrupted Healthcare.* London: Radcliffe.

Gouglas, D., Le, T. T., Henderson, K. . . . & Røttingen, J. A. (2018). Estimating the cost of vaccine development against epidemic infectious diseases. *Lancet Global Health, 6* (12): e1386–e1396.

Grassly, N. C., Pons-Salort, M., Parker, E. P., White, P. J., Ferguson, N. M., Ainslie, K., … & Cattarino, L. (2020). Comparison of molecular testing strategies for COVID-19 control: A mathematical modelling study. *The Lancet Infectious Diseases.*

Grechyna, D. (2020). Health Threats Associated with Children Lockdown in Spain during COVID-19. [online publication: March 2020]. *SSRN: 3567670.*

Greenberg, J., Koole, S. L., & Pyszczynski, T. A. (Eds.). (2014). *Handbook of Experimental Existential Psychology.* New York: Guilford Press.

Greenhalgh, T., Knight, M., Buxton, M. & Husain, L. (2020). Management of post-acute covid-19 in primary care. *British Medical Journal, 370.* [Epub ahead of print]

Gürcan, E. C. & Kahraman, Ö. E. (2020). COVID-19 in Historical Perspective: How Disaster Capitalism Fabricates a Fear-Managed World Order. Prepub: www.academia.edu

Hammond, J., Salamonson, Y., Davidson, P., Everett, B. & Andrew, S. (2007). Why do women underestimate the risk of cardiac disease? *Australian Critical Care, 20* (2): 53–9.

Haque, U. (2019). *This is How a Society Dies.* Available at https://eand.co/this-is-how-a-society-dies-35bdc3c0b854 (Accessed on 15 October 2020).

Hardt, M. D. (2015). *History of Infectious Disease Pandemics in Urban Societies.* Lanham, MD: Lexington Books.

Hardt, M. & Negri, A. (2000). *Empire.* Boston: Harvard University Press.

Haslam, S. A. (2014). Making good theory practical. *British Journal of Social Psychology, 53*: 1–20.

Hawkley, L. C. & Cacioppo, J. T. (2010). Loneliness matters: A theoretical and empirical review of consequences and mechanisms. *Annals of Behavioral Medicine, 40*(2), 218–27.

Heidegger, M. (1921/1995). *Aristotle's Metaphysics*. Bloomington, IN: Indiana University Press.

Heidegger, M. (1927/1996). *Being and Time*. London: SUNY.

Heinrich, L. M. & Gullone, E. (2006). The clinical significance of loneliness: A literature review. *Clinical Psychology Review, 26*(6), 695–718.

Henderson, D. A. & Borio, L. L. (2006). Smallpox and monkeypox. In R. L. Guerrant, D. H. Walker and P. F. Weller (Eds.) *Tropical Infectious Diseases, 2e*. London: Churchill Livingstone, pp. 621–36.

Herman, E. S. & Chomsky, N. (2010). *Manufacturing Consent*. New York: Random House.

Hoare, E., Milton, K., Foster, C. & Allender, S. (2016). The associations between sedentary behaviour and mental health among adolescents: A systematic review. *International Journal of Behavioral Nutrition and Physical Activity, 13*(1): 108–120.

Holt-Lunstad, J., Smith, T. B., Baker, M., Harris, T. & Stephenson, D. (2015). Loneliness and social isolation as risk factors for mortality: A meta-analytic review. *Perspectives on Psychological Science, 10*(2): 227–37.

Honigsbaum, M. (2019). *The Pandemic Century: One Hundred Years of Panic, Hysteria and Hubris*. Oxford: Oxford University Press.

Hoti, K., Jakupi, A., Hetemi, D., Raka, D., Hughes, J. & Desselle, S. (2020). Provision of community pharmacy services during COVID-19 pandemic: A cross sectional study of community pharmacists' experiences with preventative measures and sources of information. *International Journal of Clinical Pharmacy, 1*: 1–10.

Huang, S. K., Lindell, M. K. & Prater, C. S. (2016). Who leaves and who stays? *Environment and Behavior, 48* (8): 991–1029.

Iacobucci, G. (2020). Covid-19: Universal screening is likely to miss infected people, review finds. *BMJ: British Medical Journal (Online), 370*.

Inglesby, T. V., Nuzzo, J. B., O'Toole, T. & Henderson, D. A. (2006). Disease mitigation measures in the control of pandemic influenza. *Biosecurity and Bioterrorism, 4* (4): 366–75.

Institute of Electrical and Electronics Engineers (2005). IEEE Standard for Safety Levels with Respect to Human Exposure to Radio Frequency Electromagnetic Fields. Report.

International Commission on Non-Ionizing Radiation Protection (ICNIRP). (2009). Statement on the Guidelines for Limiting Exposure to Time-Varying Electric, Magnetic and Electromagnetic Fields. Report.

Ioannidis, J. (2020a). The infection fatality rate of COVID-19 inferred from seroprevalence data. *medRxiv*.

Ioannidis, J. P. (2020b). Coronavirus disease 2019: The harms of exaggerated information and non-evidence-based measures. *European Journal of Clinical Investigation, 50*(4), e13222.

Ioannidis, J. P. (2020c). A fiasco in the making? As the coronavirus pandemic takes hold, we are making decisions without reliable data. *Stat*: 17–30.

Ioannidis, J. P., Axfors, C. & Contopoulos-Ioannidis, D. G. (2020). Population-level COVID-19 mortality risk for non-elderly individuals overall and for non-elderly individuals without underlying diseases in pandemic epicenters. *medRxiv*.

Islam, M. S., Tonmoy, S. Khan, S. H. . . . Seale, H. (2020). *COVID-19-Related Infodemic and Its Impact on Public Health: A Global Social Media Analysis*. Preprint: www.ssrn.com

Janoff-Bulman, R. (2010). *Shattered Assumptions*. New York: Simon & Schuster.

Jefferson, T., Spencer, E., Brassey, J. & Heneghan, C. (2020). Viral cultures for COVID-19 infectivity assessment. Systematic review. *medRxiv*.

Jeong, H., Yim, H. W., Song, Y.-J., Ki, M., Min, J.-A., Cho, J. & Chae, J.-H. (2016). Mental health status of people isolated due to Middle East Respiratory Syndrome. *Epidemiology and Health*, 38: 89–101.

Jetten, J., Reicher, S. D., Haslam, S. A. & Cruwys, T. (2020). *Together Apart: The Psychology of Covid-19*. London: Sage.

Jimenez, T., Restar, A., Helm, P. J., Cross, R. I., Barath, D. & Arndt, J. (2020). Fatalism in the context of COVID-19: Perceiving coronavirus as a death sentence predicts reluctance to perform recommended preventive behaviors. *SSM-Population Health*, 11: 100615. doi:10.1016/j.ssmph.2020.100615.

Jones, E. J., Roche, C. C. & Appel, S. J. (2009). A review of the health beliefs and life-style behaviors of women with previous gestational diabetes. *Journal of Obstetric, Gynecologic & Neonatal Nursing*, 38 (5): 516–26.

Jones, O. (2015). *The Establishment: And How They Get Away With It*. London: Melville House.

Kachanoff, F., Bigman, Y., Kapsaskis, K. & Gray, K. (2020). *Measuring Two Distinct Psychological Threats of COVID-19 and Their Unique Impacts on Wellbeing and Adherence to Public Health Behaviors*. Preprint: www.medrix.org

Kamerlin, S. C. & Kasson, P. M. (2020). Managing COVID-19 spread with voluntary public-health measures. *Clinical Infectious Diseases*, ciaa864. doi:10.1093/cid/ciaa864

Kanadiya, M. K., & Sallar, A. M. (2011). Preventive behaviors, beliefs, and anxieties in relation to the swine flu outbreak among college students aged 18–24 years. *Journal of Public Health*, 19 (2), 139–145.

Keck, F. (2020). *Avian Reservoirs*. New York: Duke University.

Kelly, A. H., Keck, F. & Lynteris, C. (Eds.) (2019). *The Anthropology of Epidemics*. New York: Routledge.

Kępińska, A. P., Iyegbe, C. O., Vernon, A. C., Yolken, R., Murray, R. M. & Pollak, T. A. (2020). Schizophrenia and influenza at the centenary of the 1918–1919 Spanish influenza pandemic. *Frontiers in Psychiatry*, 11: 72.

Kilgo, D. K., Yoo, J. & Johnson, T. J. (2018). Spreading Ebola panic. *Health Communication*, 34 (8): 811–17.

Kim, J. (2020). Impact of the Perceived Threat of COVID-19 on Variety-seeking. *Australasian Marketing Journal (AMJ)*. doi: 10.1016/j.ausmj.2020.07.001.

Kim, W., Han, J. M. & Lee, K. E. (2020). Predictors of mortality in patients with COVID-19: A systematic review and meta-analysis. *Korean Journal of Clinical Pharmacy*, 30(3), 169–176.

Kirk, C. P. & Rifkin, L. S. (2020). I'll trade you diamonds for toilet paper. *Journal of Business Research*, 117: 124–31.

Kitchin, R. (2020). Civil liberties or public health, or civil liberties and public health? Using surveillance technologies to tackle the spread of COVID-19. *Space and Polity*, *1*: 1–20.

Klein, N. (2007). *The Shock Doctrine: The Rise of Disaster Capitalism*. Macmillan.

Klemm, C., Das, E. & Hartmann, T. (2016). Swine flu and hype: A systematic review of media dramatization of the H1N1 influenza pandemic. *Journal of Risk Research*, *19* (1): 1–20.

Kuhn, T. S. (2012). *The Structure of Scientific Revolutions*. Chicago: University of Chicago Press.

Lakoff, A. (2017). *Unprepared*. San Francisco: University of California.

Langgartner, D., Lowry, C. A. & Reber, S. O. (2019). Old friends, immunoregulation, and stress resilience. *European Journal of Physiology*, *471* (2): 237–69.

Larsen, E. M., Donaldson, K. & Mohanty, A. (2020). *Conspiratorial Thinking During COVID-19*. Preprint: psyarxiv.com

Lau, B. H. P., Chan, C. L. W. & Ng, S. M. (2020). *What Doesn't Kill You Makes You Stronger*. Preprint: psyarxiv.com

Lau, H., Khosrawipour, V., Kocbach, P., Mikolajczyk, R., Schubert, J., Bania, J. & Khosrawipour, T. (2020). The positive impact of lockdown in Wuhan on containing the COVID-19 outbreak in China. *Journal of Travel Medicine*, *27* (3): taaa037. doi: 10.1093/jtm/taaa037

Laurencin, C. T. & McClinton, A. (2020). The COVID-19 pandemic: A call to action to identify and address racial and ethnic disparities. *Journal of Racial and Ethnic Health Disparities*, *1*: 1–5.

Ledley, F. D., McCoy, S. S., Vaughan, G. & Cleary, E. G. (2020). Profitability of large pharmaceutical companies compared with other large public companies. *JAMA*, *323* (9): 834–43.

Leppin, A. & Aro, A. R. (2009). Risk-perceptions related to SARS and avian influenza. *International Journal of Behavioral Medicine*, *16* (1): 7–29.

Lerner, J. S. (2013). Effects of fear and anger on perceived risks. *Psychological Science*, *14*: 144–52.

Lesser, L. I., Ebbeling, C. B., Goozner, M., Wypii, D. & Ludwig, D. S. (2007). Relationship between funding source and conclusion. *PLOS*, *4* (1): e5.

Levit, M. (2020). Infection risk of COVID-19 in dentistry remains unknown: A preliminary systematic review. *Infectious Diseases in Clinical Practice*. [Epub ahead of print]

Levy, B. H. (2020). *The Virus in the Age of Madness*. Yale University Press.

Lindblom, C. E. (1959). The science of 'muddling through'. *Public Administration Review*: 79–88.

Liston, C., McEwen, B S. & Casey, B. J. (2009). Psychosocial stress reversibly disrupts prefrontal processing and attentional control. *Proceedings of National Academy of Sciences*, *106* (3): 912–17.

Liu, J. J., Bao, Y., Huang, X., Shi, J. & Lu, L. (2020). Mental health considerations for children quarantined because of COVID-19. *The Lancet Child & Adolescent Health*, *4* (5): 347–349. doi: 10.1016/S2352-4642(20)30096-1.

Long, N. N. & Khoi, B. H. (2020). An empirical study about the intention to hoard food during COVID-19 pandemic. *EURASIA*, *16* (7): em1857.

Luo, L., Fu, M., Li, Y., Hu, S., Luo, J., Chen, Z., ... & Tu, L. (2020). The potential association between common comorbidities and severity and mortality of corona-virus disease 2019: A pooled analysis. *Clinical Cardiology*. doi: 10.1002/clc.23465.

Lupton, D. (2013). *Risk*. London: Routledge.

Mahase, E. (2020a). Covid-19: Local health teams trace eight times more contacts than national service. *BMJ, 369* (m2486). doi: https://doi.org/10.1136/bmj.m2486.

Mahase, E. (2020b). Covid-19: Was the decision to delay the UK's lockdown over fears of 'behavioural fatigue' based on evidence? *British Medical Journal*. Preprint.

Marafa, L. M. & Tung, F. (2004). Changes in participation in leisure and outdoor recreation activities among Hong Kong people during the SARS outbreak. *World Leisure Journal, 46*(2): 38–47.

Marmot, M. & Wilkinson, R. (Eds.) (2005). *Social Determinants of Health*. Oxford: Oxford University Press.

Marmot, M. (2001). Inequalities in health. *New England Journal of Medicine, 345* (2): 134–5.

Martinez, C. (2020). Karl Marx in Wuhan: How Chinese socialism is defeating COVID-19. *International Critical Thought, 10* (2): 311–22.

Martinson, B. C., Anderson, M. S. & Vries, R. (2005). Scientists behaving badly. *Nature, 435* (7043): 737–8.

Mbembe, A. (2019). *Necropolitics*. Durham, NC: Duke University Press.

McGoey, L. (2015). *No Such Thing as a Free Gift: The Gates Foundation and the Price of Philanthropy*. London: Verso.

Mearns, K. & Flin, R. (1995). Risk-perception and attitudes to safety by personnel in the offshore oil and gas industry. *Journal of Loss Prevention, 8* (5): 299–305.

Menzies, R. E. & Menzies, R. G. (2020). Death anxiety in the time of COVID-19. *Cognitive Behaviour Therapist, 1*: 13.

Merleau-Ponty, M. (1982). *Phenomenology of Perception*. London: Routledge.

Mezzadri, A. (2020). A crisis like no other. *Developing Economics*. 20 April. www.developingeconomics.org

Michaels, D. (2008). *Doubt Is Their Product: How Industry's Assault on Science Threatens Your Health*. Oxford: Oxford University Press.

Milburn, M. A. & Conrad, S. D. (1998). *The Politics of Denial*. Boston: MIT Press.

Mishra, P. (2017). *Age of Anger*. London: Macmillan.

Moraes, L. J., Miranda, M. B., Loures, L. F., Mainieri, A. G. & Mármora, C. H. C. (2018). A systematic review of psychoneuroimmunology-based interventions. *Psychology, Health and Medicine, 23* (6): 635–52.

Morens, D. M., Taubenberger, J. K., Folkers, G. K. & Fauci, A. S. (2010). Pandemic influenza's 500th anniversary. *Clinical Infectious Diseases, 51* (12): 1442–4.

Mühlhoff, R. (2020). *We Need to Think Data Protection Beyond Privacy*. Preprint: www.academia.edu

Murshed, S. M. (2020). Capitalism and COVID-19: Crisis at the Crossroads. *Peace Economics, Peace Science and Public Policy* [epub-ahead-of-print]. doi:10.1515/peps-2020-0026.

Mushtaq, R., Shoib, S., Shah, T. & Mushtaq, S. (2014). Relationship between loneli-ness, psychiatric disorders and physical health? A review on the psychological aspects of loneliness. *Journal of Clinical and Diagnostic Research: JCDR, 8*(9): 1–20.

Nancy, J. L. (2020). Viral exception. *European Journal of Psychoanalysis*. March. www.journalpsychoanalysis.eu/coronavirus-and-philosophers/

Nardi, V. A. M., Teixeira, R., Ladeira, W. J. & Oliveira-Santini, F. (2020). A meta-analytic review of food safety risk-perception. *Food Control, 112*: 107089.

Nature Index (2020). Coronavirus research publishing. 17 August.

Ndugwa, K. S. & Berg-Beckhoff, G. (2015). The association between HIV/AIDS-related knowledge and perception of risk for infection. *Perspectives in Public Health, 135* (6): 299–308.

Neimeyer, R. A. (2001). *Meaning Reconstruction and the Experience of Loss.* Washington, DC: American Psychological Association.

Nelson, A. (2020). COVID-19: Capitalist and postcapitalist perspectives. *Human Geography*. doi:10.1177/1942778620937122.

Newman, M. (2020). Covid-19: Doctors' leaders warn that staff could quit and may die over lack of protective equipment. *British Medical Journal Online*: 368.

Nickson, S., Thomas, A., & Mullens-Burgess, E. (2020). Decision making in a crisis. *Institute for Government.* [Epub]

Noor, F. M. & Islam, M. M. (2020). Prevalence and associated risk factors of mortality among COVID-19 patients: A meta-analysis. *Journal of Community Health*, 1–13.

Noori, Q. (2020). *The Changes of Training Activity Level in Athletes During the COVID-19 Pandemic.* Preprint: researchgate.net

Nowicki, G. J., Ślusarska, B., Tucholska, K., Chrzan-Rodak, A. & Niedorys, B. (2020). *The Severity of Traumatic Stress Associated with COVID-19 Pandemic, Perception of Support, Sense of Security, and Sense of Meaning in Life Among Nurses.* Preprint: preprints.org

Nuki, P. & Gardner, B. (2020). Exercise Cygnus uncovered. *The Telegraph*, 28 March.

O'Campo, P. & Dunn, J. R. (2011). *Rethinking Social Epidemiology.* London: Springer.

O'Leary, M. (2004). *The First 72 Hours.* London: iUniverse.

Oleksy, T., Wnuk, A., Maison, D. & Łyś, A. (2020). Content matters. Different predictors and social consequences of general and government-related conspiracy theories on COVID-19. *Personality and Individual Differences, 168*: 110289. doi: 10.1016/j.paid.2020.110289.

Oliver, M. B., Raney, A. A. & Bryant, J. (2019). *Media Effects.* London: Routledge.

Olson, A. (2020). Lobbying expenditures of the health sector during the COVID-19 Pandemic, *Journal of General Internal Medicine.* doi: 10.1007/s11606-020-06085-6.

Omran, A. (1971). The epidemiologic transition: A theory of the epidemiology of population change. *Milbank Memorial Fund Quarterly, 49*(4): 509–38.

Oosterhoff, B. (2020). *Psychological Correlates of News Monitoring, Social Distancing, Disinfecting, and Hoarding Behaviors Among US Adolescents During the COVID-19 Pandemic.* Preprint: www.psyarxiv.com

Ornell, F., Schuch, J. B., Sordi, A. O. & Kessler, F. H. P. (2020). 'Pandemic fear' and COVID-19. *Brazilian Journal of Psychiatry, 42* (3): 232–5.

Ostry, J. D., Loungani, P. & Furcery, D. (2016). Neoliberalism: Oversold? *Finance and Development*, June.

Pedersen, A., Zachariae, R. & Bovbjerg, D. H. (2010). Influence of psychological stress on upper respiratory infection. *Psychosomatic Medicine, 72* (8): 823–32.

Pegg, D. (2020). What was exercise Cygnus? *The Guardian*, 7 May.

Penedo, F. J. & Dahn, J. R. (2005). Exercise and well-being: A review of mental and physical health benefits associated with physical activity. *Current Opinion in Psychiatry*, *18*(2), 189–193.

Pereira, E. R., Silva, R. M. C. R. A. & Dias, F. A. (2020). Psychological phases and meaning of life in times of social isolation due to the COVID-19 pandemic: A reflection in the light of Viktor Frankl. *Research, Society and Development*, *9* (5): 122953331.

Peters, G. J. Y., Ruiter, R. A., & Kok, G. (2013). Threatening communication: A critical re-analysis and a revised meta-analytic test of fear appeal theory. *Health Psychology Review*, *7*(sup1): S8–S31.

Phillips, A C., Carroll, D., Burns, V. E. & Drayson, M. (2005). Neuroticism, cortisol reactivity, and antibody response to vaccination. *Psychophysiology*, *42* (2), 232–8.

Pierre, J. (2020). Nudges against pandemics: Sweden's COVID-19 containment strategy in perspective. *Policy and Society*, *39* (3): 478–93.

Pirtle, W. N. L. (2020). Racial capitalism: A fundamental cause of novel coronavirus (COVID-19) pandemic inequities. *Health Education and Behavior*, *47*(4): 504–8. doi: 10.1177/1090198120922942.

Pormohammad, A., Ghorbani, S., Khatami, A., Razizadeh, M. H., Alborzi, E., Zarei, M., ... & Turner, R. J. (2020). Comparison of influenza type A and B with COVID-19: A global systematic review and meta-analysis on clinical, laboratory and radiographic findings. *Reviews in Medical Virology*, e2179.

Posner, G. (2020). *Pharma: Greed, Lies, and the Poisoning of America*. New York: Simon & Schuster.

Prati, G., Pietrantoni, L. & Zani, B. (2011). Compliance with recommendations for pandemic influenza H1N1 2009. *Health Education Research*, *26* (5): 761–9.

Price-Haywood, E. G., Burton, J., Fort, D. & Seoane, L. (2020). Hospitalization and mortality among black patients and white patients with Covid-19. *New England Journal of Medicine*, *382*: 2534–43.

Purdon, C. & Clark, D. A. (1994). Obsessive intrusive thoughts in nonclinical subjects. *Behaviour Research and Therapy*, *32* (4): 403–10.

Qazi, U. A. (2020). *What Went Wrong*. University Hospitals Birmingham UK. Report.

Quammen, D. (2020). *Spillover*. Rome: Adelphi.

Quick, J. D. & Fryer, B. (2018). *The End of Epidemics*. London: St. Martin's Press.

Ratcliff, K. S. (2017). *The Social Determinants of Health: Looking Upstream*. London: John Wiley.

Reiss, K. & Bhakdi, S. (2020). *Corona, False Alarm?*. London: Chelsea Green Publishing.

Reissman, D. B., Watson, P. J., Klomp, R. W., Tanielian, T. L. & Prior, S. D. (2006). Pandemic influenza preparedness. *Journal of Homeland Security Emergency Management*. *3*: 1–24.

Rettie, H. & Daniels, J. (2020). Coping and tolerance of uncertainty. *American Psychologist*. Pre-print online.

Richards, D. & Boudnik, K. (2020). Neil Ferguson's Imperial model could be the most devastating software mistake of all time. *The Telegraph*, 17 May.

Rimmer, A. (2020). Covid-19: Impact of long-term symptoms will be profound, warns BMA. *British Medical Journal*, *370*: 3218.

Romano, J. L. (2020). Politics of prevention. *Journal of Prevention and Health Promotion*. Pre-print online.

Rosanvallon, P. (2013). La Légitimité Démocratique: Impartialité, Réflexivité, Proximité. Paris: Seuil.

Rosanvallon, P. (2018). *Good Government: Democracy Beyond Elections*. Cambridge: Harvard University Press.

Rosenfeld, D. L. & Tomiyama, A. J. (2020). *Can a Pandemic Make People More Socially Conservative?* Pre-print: www.psyarxiv.com

Rovelli.C. (2018). *Reality Is Not What It Seems*. London: Penguin.

Saad-Filho, A. (2020). From COVID-19 to the End of Neoliberalism. *Critical Sociology*. Pre-print online.

Sabeti, P. & Salahi, L. (2018). *Outbreak Culture: The Ebola Crisis and the Next Epidemic*. London: Harvard University Press.

Sadati, A. K. B, Lankarani, M. H. & Bagheri-Lankarani, K. (2020). Risk society, global vulnerability and fragile resilience: Sociological view on the Coronavirus outbreak. *Shiraz, 21*(4): e102263. doi: 10.5812/semj.102263.

Salkovskis, P. M., Forrester, E. & Richards, C. (1998). Cognitive–behavioural approach to understanding obsessional thinking. *British Journal of Psychiatry, 173* (S35): 53–63.

Sallam, M., Dababseh, D., Yaseen, A., Al-Haidar, A., Ababneh, N. A., Bakri, F. G. & Mahafzah, A. (2020). Conspiracy beliefs are associated with lower knowledge and higher anxiety levels. *International Journal of Environmental Research and Public Health, 17* (14): 4915.

San Juan, D. M. (2020). *Responding to COVID-19 Through Socialist Measures*. Preprint: www.ssrn.com

Sandman, P. M. (1987). Risk communication. *EPA, 13*: 21.

Sandman, P. M. (1993). *Responding to Community Outrage*. New York: AIHA.

Satici, B., Saricali, M., Satici, S. A. & Griffiths, M. D. (2020). Intolerance of uncertainty and mental wellbeing. *International Journal of Mental Health and Addiction*. Pre-print online.

Savage, D. A. (2019). Towards a complex model of disaster behaviour. *Disasters, 43* (4): 771–98.

Savasta, A. M. (2004). HIV: Associated transmission risks in adults. *Journal of the Association of Nurses in AIDS Care, 15* (1): 50–9.

Schaller, M. & Park, J. H. (2011). The behavioral immune system. *Current Directions in Psychological Science, 20*: 99–103.

Schlegel, R. J., Hicks, J. A., Arndt, J. & King, L. A. (2009). Thine own self: True self-concept accessibility and meaning in life. *Journal of Personality and Social Psychology, 96* (2): 473.

Schulenberg, S. E., Drescher, C. F. & Baczwaski, B. J. (2014). Perceived meaning and disaster mental health: A role for logotherapy in clinical-disaster psychology. In A. Batthyany & P. Russo-Netzer (Eds.), *Meaning in Positive and Existential Psychology*. New York: Springer, pp. 251–67.

Schwab, K. & Malleret, T. (2020). *COVID-19: The Great Reset*. Cologne and Geneva: World Economic Forum.

Scoones, I. & Stirling, A. (2020). *The Politics of Uncertainty: Challenges of Transformation*. New York: Taylor & Francis.

Segerstrom, S. C. & Miller, G. E. (2004). Psychological stress and the human immune system: A meta-analytic study of 30 years of inquiry. *Psychological Bulletin, 130*(4): 601–10.

Selye, H. (1950). Stress and the general adaptation syndrome. *British Medical Journal, 1* (4667): 1383.

Sergent, K. & Stajkovic, A. D. (2020). Women's leadership is associated with fewer deaths during the COVID-19 crisis. *Journal of Applied Psychology, 8*: 771–81.

Serlin, I. & Cannon, J. T. (2004). *Living with Terror, Working with Trauma.* New York: Springer.

Severance, E. G., Dickerson, F. B., Viscidi, R. P. . . . & Yolken, R. H. (2011). Coronavirus immunoreactivity in individuals with a recent onset of psychotic symptoms. *Schizophrenia Bulletin, 37* (1): 101–7.

Shamasunder, S., Holmes, S. M., Goronga, T., Carrasco, H., Katz, E., Frankfurter, R. & Keshavjee, S. (2020). COVID-19 reveals weak health systems by design. *Global Public Health, 1*: 1–7.

Shanahan, L., Steinhoff, A., Bechtiger, L. . . . & Eisner, M. (2020). Emotional distress in young adults during the COVID-19 pandemic. *Psychological Medicine, 1*: 1–10.

Shao, W. & Hao, F. (2020). Confidence in political leaders can slant risk-perceptions of COVID-19 in a highly polarized environment. *Social Science and Medicine, 261*: 113235.

Sharma, M., Yadav, K., Yadav, N. & Ferdinand, K. C. (2017). Zika virus pandemic – analysis of Facebook. *American Journal of Infection Control, 45* (3): 301–2.

Shattuck, E. C. & Muehlenbein, M. P. (2016). Towards an integrative picture of human sickness behavior. *Brain, Behavior, and Immunity, 57*: 255–62.

Singer, M. (2009). *Introduction to Syndemics.* New York: John Wiley.

Singh R. & Adhikari, R. (2020). Age-structured impact of social distancing on the COVID-19 epidemic in India. *ArXiv.*

Slovic, P. (2001). *Smoking.* London: Sage.

Smith, J. G. (2020). Responding to coronavirus pandemic. *Interface, 1*: 1–8.

Sobande, F. (2020). 'We're all in this together': Commodified notions of connection, care and community in brand responses to COVID-19. *European Journal of Cultural Studies, 1*: 1367549420932294. doi:10.1177/1367549420932294

Solomon, S., Greenberg, J. & Pyszczynski, T. (2015). *The Worm at the Core: On the Role of Death in Life.* New York: Random House.

Sotiris, P. (2020). Against Agamben: Is a democratic biopolitics possible? *Viewpoint.* 20 March. www.viewpointmag.com/2

Stephany, F., Stoehr, N., Darius, P., Neuhauser, L., Teutloff, O. & Braesemann, F. (2020). Which industries are most severely affected by the COVID-19 pandemic? A data-mining approach to identify industry-specific risks in real-time. *MyIDEAS: April 2020.*

Stirling, A. (2008). Science, precaution, and the politics of technological risk: Converging implications in evolutionary and social scientific perspectives. *Annals of the New York Academy of Sciences, 1128*(1), 95–110.

Streeck, H. (2020). Einzelne Ubertragungen im Supermarkt sind nicht das Problem. *Zeit Online.* 6 April.

Stroebe, M., Schut, H. & Boerner, K. (2017). Cautioning health-care professionals. *OMEGA, 74* (4): 455–73.

Sun, P., Lu, X., Xu, C., Sun, W. & Pan, B. (2020). Understanding of COVID-19 based on current evidence. *Journal of Medical Virology, 92* (6): 548–51.

Surkova, E., Nikolayevskyy, V. & Drobniewski, F. (2020). False-positive COVID-19 results: Hidden problems and costs. *The Lancet Respiratory Medicine.* [Epub ahead of print]

Swami, V. & Barron, D. (2020). *Analytic Thinking, Rejection of Coronavirus Conspiracy Theories, and Compliance with Mandated Social-distancing.* Pre-print: osf.io

Tabri, N., Hollingshead, S. & Wohl, M. (2020). *Framing Covid-19 as an Existential Threat Predicts Anxious Arousal and Prejudice Towards Chinese People.* Pre-print: www.psyarxiv.com

Tang, L., Bie, B., Park, S. E. & Zhi, D. (2018). Social media and outbreaks of emerging infectious diseases. *American Journal of Infection Control, 46* (9): 962–72.

Tangney, J. P. & Dearing, R. L. (2003). *Shame and Guilt.* London: Guilford Press.

Tasnim, S., Hossain, M. M. & Mazumder, H. (2020). Impact of rumors and misinformation on COVID-19. *Journal of Preventive Medicine and Public Health, 53* (3): 171–4.

Taylor, S. (2019). *The Psychology of Pandemics.* Cambridge: Cambridge Scholars.

Tooher, R., Collins, J. E., Street, J. M., Braunack-Mayer A. & Marshall, H. (2013). Community knowledge, behaviours and attitudes about the 2009 H1N1 influenza pandemic. *Influenza and Other Respiratory Viruses, 7* (6): 1316–27.

Torjeson, I. (2020). Covid-19 pre-purchasing: Sensible or selfish? *British Medical Journal, 370*: 3226.

Torrey, E. F., Miller, J., Rawlings, R. & Yolken, R. H. (1997). Seasonality of births in schizophrenia and bipolar disorder. *Schizophrenia Research, 28* (1): 1–38.

Trnka, R. & Lorencova, R. (2020). Fear, anger, and media-induced trauma during the outbreak of COVID-19 in the Czech Republic. *Psychological Trauma, 12* (5): 546–9.

Trumbo, C. W. (2002). Information processing and risk-perception. *Journal of Communication, 52*: 367–82.

Trzebiński, J., Cabański, M. & Czarnecka, J. Z. (2020). Reaction to the COVID-19 pandemic. *Journal of Loss and Trauma, 1*: 1–14.

Tull, M. T., Barbano, A. C., Scamaldo, K. M., Richmond, J. R., Edmonds, K. A., Rose, J. P. & Gratz, K. L. (2020) The prospective influence of COVID-19 affective risk assessments and intolerance of uncertainty on later dimensions of health anxiety. *Journal of Anxiety Disorders, 75*: 102290. doi:10.1016/j.janxdis.2020.102290.

Tyner, J. & Rice, S. (2020). Meaningful life in the time of Corona-economics. *Dialogues in Human Geography, 10*(2):116–119. doi:10.1177/2043820620934921.

Ufearoh, A. U. (2020). COVID-19 Pandemic as an Existential Problem: An African Perspective. *Filosofia Theoretica, 9*(1): 97–112.

Ulmer, R. R., Sellnow, T. L. & Seeger, M. W. (2017). *Effective Crisis Communication: Moving from Crisis to Opportunity.* London: Sage.

Um, N. (2020). Biopower, mediascapes, and the politics of fear in the age of COVID-19. *City and Society, 1*: 1–10.

Uscinski, J. E. (2020). *Conspiracy Theories: A Primer.* Rowman & Littlefield Publishers.

Uscinski, J. E., Enders, A. M., Klofstad, C., Seelig, M., Funchion, J., Everett, C., … & Murthi, M. (2020). Why do people believe COVID-19 conspiracy theories? *Harvard Kennedy School Misinformation Review, 1*(3). [Epub ahead of print]

Vali, M., Mirahmadizadeh, A., Maleki, Z., Goudarzi, F., Abedinzade, A. & Ghaem, H. (2020). The impact of quarantine, isolation, and social distancing on COVID-19 prevention: A systematic review. *Journal of Health Sciences & Surveillance System*, *8*(4), 138–50.

Van Leeuwen, F. & Petersen, M. B. (2018). The behavioral immune system is designed to avoid infected individuals, not outgroups. *Evolution and Human Behavior*, *39*: 226–34.

Vandenbroucke, J. P. (2006). Case reports of suspected adverse drug reactions: Case reports were dismissed too quickly. *BMJ*, *332*(7539): 488–500.

VanderWeele, T. J (2020). Challenges estimating total lives lost in COVID-19 decisions. *JAMA*, *324* (5): 445–6.

Vaughan, E. & Tinker, T. (2009). Effective health risk communication about pandemic influenza for vulnerable populations. *American Journal of Public Health*, *99* (S2): S324–S332.

Vazqueza, C., Valientea, C., García, F. E., Contrerasa, A., Peinadoa, V., Truchartea, A. & Bentallc, R. P. (2020). *Post-traumatic Growth and Stress-related Responses During the COVID-19 Pandemic.* Pre-print: osf.io

Vernon, S. W. (1999). Risk-perception and Risk Communication for Cancer Screening Behaviors, *JNCI Monographs*, *25*: 101–19.

Vos, J. (2005). Het migrant-zijn van Turkse en Marokkaanse immigranten in Nederland: niet-meer en nog-niet. Een fenomenologische analyse. University Leiden, Faculty of Philosophy.

Vos, J. (2011). *Opening the Psychological Black Box in Genetic Counseling.* Enschede: Gildeprintz.

Vos, J. (2014). Meaning and existential givens in the lives of cancer patients: A philosophical perspective on psycho-oncology. *Palliative & Supportive Care*, *13*(4): 885–900.

Vos, J. (2016). Working with meaning in life in chronic or life-threatening disease: A review of its relevance and the effectiveness of meaning-centred therapies. In P. Russo-Netzer, S. E. Schulenberg and A. Batthyany (Eds.) *Clinical Perspectives on Meaning.* London: Springer, pp. 171–200.

Vos, J. (2018). *Meaning in Life: An Evidence-Based Handbook for Practitioners.* London: Macmillan.

Vos, J. (2020). *The Economics of Meaning in Life: From Capitalist Life Syndrome to Meaning-Oriented Economy.* Colorado Springs: CO: University Professors Press.

Vos, J. (2020a). The mental health impact of COVID-19: A meta-analysis. Under review. Pre-publication at *PsyRevX*.

Vos, J. (2020b). Risk-perception related to COVID-19: A meta-analysis. Under review.

Vos, J. (2020c). Risk-perception and psychological impact of COVID-19: Findings from an international survey. Under review.

Vos, J. & Vitali, D. (2018). The effects of psychological meaning-centered therapies on quality of life and psychological stress: A metaanalysis. *Supportive Care*, *16*(5), 608–32.

Vos, J., Roberts, R. & Davies, J. (2019). *Mental Health in Crisis.* London: Sage.

Vos, J. Menko, F., Jansen, A. M. . . . Tibben, A. (2011). A whisper-game perspective on the family communication of DNA-test results. *Familial Cancer*, *10* (1): 87–96.

Vosoughi, S., Roy, D. & Aral, S. (2018). The spread of true and false news online. *Science, 359* (6380): 1146–51.

Warren, E. A., Paterson, P., Schulz, W. S., Lees, S., Eakle, R., Stadler, J. & Larson, H. J. (2018). Risk-perception and the influence on uptake and use of biomedical prevention interventions. *PloS one, 13* (6): e0198680.

Watson, J., Whiting, P. F. & Brush, J. E. (2020). Interpreting a covid-19 test result. *British Medical Journal, 369*[Epub].

Watts, A. (1951). *The Wisdom of Insecurity.* London: Vintage.

Wells, K. & Lurgi, M. (2020). COVID-19 containment policies through time may cost more lives at metapopulation level. *medRxiv.*

Westlund, O. & Weibull, L. (2013). Generation, life course and news media use in Sweden 1986–2011. *Northern Lights, 11* (1): 147–73.

Westoby, P. & Harris, V. (2020). Community development 'yet-to-come' during and post COVID-19 pandemic. *Community Development Journal,* 1–17. doi: 10.1093/cdj/bsaa026.

White, A. I. (2020). Historical linkages: Epidemic threat, economic risk, and xenophobia. *The Lancet, 395* (10232): 1250–1.

Wolfe, N. (2011). *The Viral Storm.* London: Macmillan.

Wong, P. (2020). *Made for Resilience and Happiness.* Toronto: Independent Publishing.

Wu, Y., Li, H. & Li, S. (2020). *Clinical Determinants of the Severity of Coronavirus Disease 2019 (COVID-19): A Systematic Review and Meta-Analysis.* doi: 10.21203/rs.3.rs-56852/v1.

Xiang, Y. T., Zhao, Y. J., Liu, Z. H., Li, X. H., Zhao, N., Cheung, T. & Ng, C. H. (2020). The COVID-19 outbreak and psychiatric hospitals in China. *International Journal of Biological Sciences, 16* (10): 1741.

Xiao, K., Zhai, J., Feng, Y. . . . Zhang, Z. (2020). Isolation of SARS-CoV-2-related coronavirus from Malayan pangolins. *Nature, 1*: 1–4.

Xu, Y., Li, Z. X., Yu, W. J. . . . Chen, J. (2020). *Impact of the COVID-19 Pandemic on Willingness to Adopt Healthy Dietary Habits in China.* Pre-print: researchsquare.com

Yancy, C. W. (2020). COVID-19 and African Americans. *JAMA, 323* (19): 1891–2.

Yang, E. V. & Glaser, R. (2000). Stress-induced immunomodulation. *Biomedicine and Pharmacotherapy, 54* (5): 245–50.

Yang, M. (2020). Resilience and meaning-making amid the COVID-19 epidemic in China. *Journal of Humanistic Psychology, 60*(5): 662–71. doi:10.1177/0022167820929215.

Yao, H., Chen, J. H. & Xu, Y. F. (2020). Patients with mental health disorders in the COVID-19 epidemic. *Lancet Psychiatry, 7* (4): e21.

Yilmazkuday, H. (2020). Coronavirus Effects on the US Unemployment: Evidence from Google Trends. *SSRN: 3559860.*

Yu, Y. & Li, B. (2020). Effects of mindfulness and meaning in life on psychological distress in Chinese university students during the COVID-19 epidemic. *Asian Journal of Psychiatry, 53*: 102211. doi: 10.1016/j.ajp.2020.102211.

Yu, Y., Yu, Y. & Lin, Y. (2020). Cross-lagged analysis of the interplay between meaning in life and positive mental health during the COVID-19 epidemic. *Asian Journal of Psychiatry, 54*: 102278. doi:10.1016/j.ajp.2020.102278.

Zheng, Y., Goh, E. & Wen, J. (2020). The effects of misleading media reports about COVID-19 on Chinese tourists' mental health: A perspective article. *Anatolia, 31* (2): 337–40.

Zhong, B., Huang, Y. & Liu, Q. (2020). Mental health toll from the coronavirus: Social media usage reveals Wuhan residents' depression and secondary trauma in the COVID-19 outbreak. *Computers in Human Behavior, 1:* 106524.

Zhou, P., Yang, X. L., Wang, X. G. . . . Chen, H. D. (2020). A pneumonia outbreak associated with a new coronavirus of probable bat origin. *Nature, 579* (7798): 270–3.

Zhu, X., Levasseur, P. R., Michaelis, K. A., Burfeind, K. G. & Marks, D. L. (2016). A distinct brain pathway links viral RNA exposure to sickness behavior. *Scientific Reports, 6:* 29885.

INDEX

Page numbers in **bold** indicate tables.

Lightning Source UK Ltd.
Milton Keynes UK
UKHW011425131021
392123UK00002B/172